THE ULTIMATE SUPPLEMENT GUIDE FOR PERFORMANCE AND HEALTH:

Optimize Your Body and Mind with Essential Supplements

The Ultimate Supplement Guide for Performance and Health: Optimize Your Body and Mind with Essential Supplements

Description

Dive into this comprehensive supplement guide, designed to help you understand, select, and make the most of supplements that support both physical and mental performance. From elite athletes to individuals seeking to enhance overall well-being, this book offers a well-researched, accessible perspective on how proper supplementation can optimize your life. Explore the benefits, recommended doses, and scientific evidence behind each supplement; discover when and why to consider them; and learn how to integrate them into your daily routine to achieve your goals naturally and effectively.

With a focus on personalization, this book also addresses the importance of tailoring supplementation to your specific needs, considering factors like exercise, nutrition, rest, and overall health. Featuring practical advice, informational tables, and an inclusive approach (including vegan and plant-based options), this guide is your essential reference for transforming your energy and health from the inside out.

Index

1. **Introduction to Supplementation**

   - **What is supplementation, and why is it important?**
   - **Evolution of supplements in health and fitness**
   - **The role of supplements: necessity or complement?**
     How to use this guide and personalize your supplementation

2. **Fundamental Criteria for Selecting Supplements**

   - **Quality assessment: how to choose safe and effective supplements**
   - **The importance of bioavailability: maximizing absorption and effects**
   - **Scientific evidence and supporting data: how to read and understand studies**
   - **Supplementation by specific goals: performance, health, longevity, mental wellness**
     Considerations for vegans and vegetarians: plant-based sources and alternatives

3. **Essential Supplements for Health and Performance**

   - **Protein (Bonus protein shake and banana bread recipes)**

     - **What it is and how it functions in the body**
     - **Protein sources and their benefits**
     - **Recommended doses based on goals (maintenance, muscle gain, etc.)**
     - **Plant-based and vegan options**
     - **Tips for optimizing absorption and timing**
     - **Potential side effects and contraindications**

   - **Caffeine**

     - **Mechanism of action and performance effects**
     - **Benefits and precautions of caffeine use**
     - **Recommended doses and timing**
     - **Caffeine and exercise: what studies say**
       Caffeine-free alternatives and plant-based options

   - **Creatine**

     - **Creatine as a key supplement for strength and performance**
     - **Mechanism of action and benefits**
     - **Dosage, types of creatine, and how to choose the best option**
     - **Scientific evidence on safety and efficacy**

Considerations for women, vegans, and older adults

- **Vitamin D**

  - Importance of vitamin D for immune health and performance
  - Specific benefits for bones, muscles, and general health
  - Doses based on levels and sun exposure
  - When and how to supplement (seasonality, deficiencies)
  - Vegan alternatives and dietary sources

- **Magnesium**

  - Role of magnesium in performance, sleep, and recovery
  - Recommended doses and types of magnesium
  - Is supplementation necessary? Groups at risk of deficiency
  - Tips to maximize absorption (useful combinations)
  - Side effects and precautions

- **Vitamin B12**

  - Fundamental role of vitamin B12 in energy and metabolism
  - Doses and recommendations for vegans and vegetarians
  - How to detect deficiencies and when to supplement
  - Plant-based sources and practical recommendations
  - Consequences of deficiency and side effects of supplementation

- **Omega-3**

  - Effects of omega-3 on the brain, heart, and muscle recovery
  - Recommended doses and main sources (animal and plant)
  - Comparison between fish oil, algae, and other plant oils
  - Scientific evidence and recent studies
  - Ideal supplementation for vegans and practical options

- **Coenzyme Q10**

  - Benefits of CoQ10 for energy and cardiovascular health
  - Mechanism of action and optimal doses
  - Who should consider supplementation?
  - Interactions and precautions with other supplements or medications
  - Vegan sources and key scientific data

- **Melatonin**

  - Melatonin's role in sleep regulation
  - Dosage, timing, and potential side effects
  - Recommendations for jet lag and sleep disorders
  - Natural alternatives and precautions
  - Scientific evidence and its relationship to sleep quality

- **Ashwagandha**

  - Natural adaptogen and its effects on stress and energy
  - Recommended doses and proven benefits
  - Side effects and contraindications
  - Ashwagandha alternatives for vegans and natural consumers
  - Studies on its role in exercise and recovery

4. **Practical Supplementation Guide by Personal Needs**

   - How to personalize your supplementation plan
   - Supplements by goals: performance, mental health, longevity
   - Recommendations for teenagers, adults, and seniors
   - Quick reference tables by supplement type and dose

5. **Tips to Enhance Supplementation Effects**

   - The relationship between exercise, diet, and rest
   - Useful combinations and synergistic supplements
   - Circadian rhythms and the best timing for each supplement
   - Habits to optimize physical and mental performance

6. **Motivation and Mindset Strategies to Achieve Your Goals**

   - The importance of a positive mindset
   - Setting SMART goals
   - Visualization and success mindset
   - Self-motivation techniques
   - Overcoming obstacles and reframing thoughts

7. **Supplementation in Recovery and Injury Prevention**

   - Natural anti-inflammatory supplements: Omega-3, Turmeric, and Resveratrol
   - Joint health supplements: Glucosamine, Chondroitin, and Collagen
   - Muscle recovery: The importance of BCAAs, Protein, and Magnesium in post-workout recovery

- o Additional recovery strategies
- o How to monitor recovery: signs of overtraining and preventing common injuries

8. **Nutrition and Supplementation for Cognitive Performance**

- o The connection between nutrition and cognitive performance
- o Supplements for concentration and memory: Omega-3, Ginkgo Biloba, Ashwagandha, and Rhodiola
- o Essential micronutrients for brain health: Importance of B Vitamins, Magnesium, and Zinc
- o Tips to optimize cognitive performance
- o Balanced nutrition for brain health: Sample day of eating focused on mental well-being

9. **Meal Planning and Preparation to Support Supplementation**

- o How to combine supplements with food to optimize absorption
- o Weekly meal planning
- o Practical recipes for health and performance
- o Tips for meal prep
- o Healthy snack options to boost energy and recovery

10. **Supplementation for Different Types of Training**

- o Strength and muscle endurance training
- o Endurance training (cardio, long-distance)
- o HIIT and CrossFit
- o Yoga, Pilates, and flexibility sports
- o Examples of supplementation by training type: recommended doses and timing

11. **Myths and Realities about Supplementation**

- o Popular supplements: myth or reality?
- o What science supports versus popular beliefs
- o How to avoid falling for misleading marketing and make informed purchases

12. **Final Considerations and Supplementation Planning**

- o How to track your results
- o Recommendations for starting supplementation safely
- o How to adapt your supplementation over time
- o Reliable sources of information and current studies
- o Frequently asked questions

13. Additional Resources and Bibliography

- o **Scientific references and recommended readings**
- o **Websites and apps for monitoring and optimization**
- o **Books and articles for deeper exploration**

Introduction to Supplementation

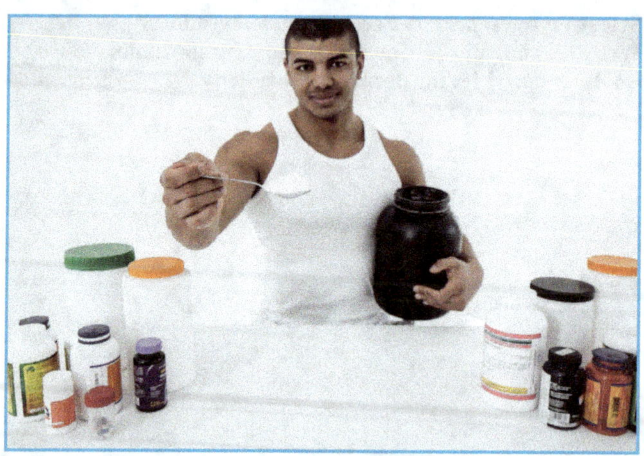

What is Supplementation and Why is it Important?

Supplementation refers to the use of products designed to provide specific nutrients or bioactive compounds that may not be available in sufficient quantities through a conventional diet. These supplements include vitamins, minerals, amino acids, fatty acids, plant extracts, and other compounds that support health, athletic performance, recovery, and general well-being.

Modern lifestyles, marked by stress, fast food, and exposure to unfavorable environmental factors, can lead to nutritional deficiencies or the inability to meet our needs solely through diet. This is where supplementation becomes a valuable tool. Proper supplementation can:**Cubrir deficiencias nutricionales:** Cuando la dieta diaria no es suficiente para satisfacer todos los requerimientos de nutrientes.

Address Nutritional Deficiencies: When a daily diet is insufficient to meet all nutrient requirements.

Optimize Physical and Mental Performance: Supplements like caffeine, creatine, and omega-3 have proven effects in improving both physical activity and cognitive function.

Support Recovery and Rest: Supplements such as melatonin, magnesium, and ashwagandha help regulate sleep and stress, both essential for effective recovery.

Prevent or Treat Specific Health Conditions: Certain supplements can help reduce disease risk or support the management of specific conditions, like vitamin D for bone health or omega-3 for cardiovascular health.

The key to successful supplementation lies in personalizing it according to your needs, goals, and lifestyle. It's not about "taking something for the sake of it" but about thoughtfully assessing what could benefit you and at what dose, based on science and personal or professional evaluation.

The history of supplementation goes back to ancient times, when herbs and natural extracts were used for medicinal and strengthening purposes. However, the modern concept of supplements began in the 20th century with the development of the first synthetic vitamins, like vitamin C and the B vitamins. Since then, supplements have evolved, diversifying and specializing.

In the 1970s and 1980s, athletes began using supplements to enhance performance and recovery, especially with protein powders and essential amino acids. Over recent decades, the field of supplementation has expanded exponentially, supported by a growing research base and increased interest in holistic well-being. Today, supplements are formulated to meet very specific needs: from improving memory and reducing stress to supporting metabolic and cardiovascular health.

Supplementation has shifted from being an athlete-exclusive practice to becoming a tool for preventive health and general wellness. Modern supplements are designed not only to "fill gaps" but also to optimize different aspects of modern life, where the balance between nutrition, rest, and exercise is increasingly challenging to achieve solely through diet.

When discussing supplementation, it's important to understand its role in health and performance. While supplements can offer significant benefits, they should not replace a balanced, healthy diet. Well-structured nutrition remains the fundamental base of any healthy lifestyle.

Supplementation by Necessity: In some cases, supplementation is almost essential. Individuals with nutritional deficiencies, those following restrictive diets (like vegans or vegetarians), or those with specific health conditions (e.g., anemia or chronic fatigue syndrome) greatly benefit from certain supplements. These supplements help address deficiencies that can't be corrected solely through dietary changes.

Supplementation as a Complement: For individuals following a balanced diet, supplements can be a tool to further optimize health and performance. For example, athletes needing more protein, those looking to improve recovery with magnesium or melatonin, or those seeking an extra dose of antioxidants to counteract stress.

It's essential to remember that supplementation is most effective when it's integrated into a healthy lifestyle. Supplements do not compensate for an imbalanced diet, a sedentary lifestyle, or lack of rest.

How to Use This Guide and Personalize Your Supplementation

This guide is designed to provide you with a comprehensive overview of the key supplements you can incorporate into your life, whether to improve physical performance, support mental health, or strengthen your immune system. Throughout the book, you'll find detailed information on each supplement, including:

Description and Function: Understand each supplement's nature, composition, and how it works in the body.

Science-backed Benefits: We'll explore scientific studies and data supporting the benefits and uses of each supplement.

Recommended Dosages: Each supplement includes suggested doses based on scientific evidence and expert recommendations. We'll also address how to adjust dosages according to your goals and profile.

Consumption Recommendations: Discover the best time of day to take each supplement and how to combine them for optimal results.

Precautions and Side Effects: Learn about possible side effects and contraindications, helping you make informed decisions.

Vegan Alternatives and Plant-based Options: We've included plant-based alternatives and options for those following a vegan diet, facilitating ethical and accessible supplementation for everyone.

As you read this guide, consider that not every supplement is a universal recommendation. Not everyone needs the same supplementation, and what works for one person may not be effective or necessary for another. Use this guide as a tool to understand which supplements might be useful in your specific situation, and consult a professional if you have specific questions or health conditions that require supervision.

How to Personalize Your Supplementation

Define Your Goals: Are you looking to enhance performance, gain muscle mass, reduce stress, or simply maintain good health? Clarifying what you want to achieve is the first step.

Assess Your Diet and Lifestyle: If you follow a complete and balanced diet, you may not need many supplements. However, if you follow a restrictive diet or have limitations on consuming certain foods, additional support may be necessary.

Consider Your Specific Needs: Age, gender, activity level, and health status influence supplementation needs. For example, older adults may benefit from supplements like vitamin D and magnesium, while athletes often require additional protein and creatine.

Review the Scientific Evidence: Throughout this book, we include data from scientific studies. It's helpful to know there are different levels of evidence, and not all supplements are supported equally.

Listen to Your Body: If you try a supplement and observe improvements, that's a positive sign. If, on the other hand, you experience discomfort or side effects, it may not be the right supplement for you.

Fundamental Criteria for Selecting Supplements

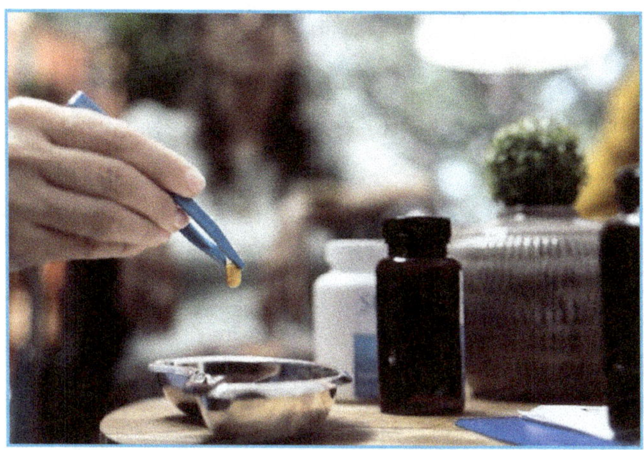

The supplement industry has grown exponentially in recent decades, and today there is an enormous variety of products available. However, not all supplements are equal in terms of quality, effectiveness, and safety. Before adding a supplement to your routine, it is essential to make a careful and well-informed selection, considering key aspects like quality, bioavailability, and supporting scientific evidence. In this chapter, we'll examine each of these criteria to help you choose supplements that can genuinely contribute to your health and performance goals.

Quality Assessment: How to Choose Safe and Effective Supplements

The quality of a supplement is one of the most critical factors, as it determines its effectiveness and safety. Low-quality supplements may contain contaminants, have fewer active ingredients than claimed, or include unnecessary additives. Here are some aspects to help you evaluate a supplement's quality:

Verify Purity and Potency: Choose supplements that clearly indicate the exact amount of each ingredient on the label and have undergone purity testing. Potency means that the supplement contains the optimal level of active ingredient necessary to be effective.

Look for Quality Certifications: Third-party certifications, such as NSF International, USP (U.S. Pharmacopeia), and GMP (Good Manufacturing Practices), indicate that the supplement has been verified by an external organization for purity, potency, and absence of contaminants.

Avoid Unnecessary Additives: Some supplements include fillers, colorants, preservatives, and other additives that may be unnecessary or harmful. Opt for products with as few additional ingredients as possible.

Choose Bioactive Forms: Some supplements are available in different chemical forms, and not all are absorbed equally. For instance, vitamin B12 in the form of methylcobalamin is more bioavailable than cyanocobalamin. Select the form of each supplement with the highest bioavailability and scientific backing.

The Importance of Bioavailability: Maximizing Absorption and Effects

Bioavailability refers to the body's ability to absorb and utilize a supplement once ingested. A supplement can contain high-quality ingredients, but if it's poorly absorbed, its benefits will be minimal. Here's how to consider bioavailability in your choices:

Supplement Forms and Absorption: Some nutrients are better absorbed in liquid or liposomal (fat-encapsulated) form, like vitamin D and Coenzyme Q10, while others, like magnesium, are better absorbed in specific forms (magnesium citrate vs. magnesium oxide). Research the ideal form for each supplement.

Use Co-factors to Enhance Absorption: The absorption of some nutrients improves when taken alongside other co-factors. For example, vitamin D absorption improves with vitamin K2 and healthy fats, while iron is better absorbed with vitamin C.

Avoid Interference with Other Nutrients or Medications: Some supplements can interfere with the absorption of other nutrients. For instance, calcium can inhibit the absorption of iron and zinc. Consider possible interactions and consult a professional if you're taking multiple supplements or medications.

Scientific Evidence and Supporting Data: How to Read and Understand Studies

Scientific evidence is essential in determining if a supplement truly delivers the promised benefits. Here are some steps to interpret and evaluate the scientific evidence for a supplement:

Review Human Studies: Animal or laboratory studies do not always translate to effects in humans. Look for studies conducted on people, ideally in contexts similar to your own (age, gender, lifestyle).

Analyze Study Size and Duration: Studies with more participants and of longer duration tend to provide more reliable results. A supplement may show effects in small studies, but these may not be replicated in larger, more robust studies.

Look for Randomized, Double-Blind Studies: Controlled and double-blind studies are the gold standard in scientific research, as they minimize bias. If a supplement has been evaluated under these conditions, confidence in its benefits increases.

Consult Systematic Reviews and Meta-Analyses: These types of research aggregate and analyze data from multiple studies, offering a broader perspective on the effectiveness of a supplement. Meta-analyses, in particular, provide an objective overview of whether a supplement is genuinely effective.

Consider the Source of Information: Be cautious of studies funded by the same companies that manufacture the supplement, as they may have an interest bias. It's preferable to rely on independent or peer-reviewed research.

Supplementation by Specific Goals: Performance, Health, Longevity, Mental Wellness

Supplementation goals vary greatly from person to person, and identifying your specific goals can help you select the right supplements. Here's a breakdown of common supplements based on primary goals:

Physical Performance: Performance-focused supplements aim to enhance strength, endurance, and recovery. Examples include creatine, caffeine, and BCAAs (branched-chain amino acids), which are useful for those seeking extra support in training and muscle growth.

General Health: This approach focuses on maintaining an optimal health state, supporting the immune system, and reducing the risk of deficiencies. Supplements like vitamin D, magnesium, omega-3, and probiotics are suitable for individuals looking to improve or maintain daily wellness.

Longevity and Disease Prevention: For those aiming to prevent illness and improve long-term quality of life, some supplements can play a preventive role. Coenzyme Q10 and antioxidants (such as vitamins E and C) can help combat cellular aging and support cardiovascular health.

Mental Wellness and Stress Reduction: Supplementation can be helpful for those seeking to improve mood and reduce stress. Supplements like ashwagandha, magnesium, and B vitamins have been studied for their ability to reduce stress, improve sleep quality, and support mental health.

Considerations for Vegans and Vegetarians: Plant-Based Alternatives and Sources

Supplementation for vegans and vegetarians requires special attention, as some traditional sources of essential nutrients (like omega-3 from fish oil or vitamin D3 from lanolin) are not suitable for this group. Here are the most important options and considerations:

Vitamin B12: B12 is an essential vitamin found only in animal sources. For vegans and vegetarians, supplementation is crucial. It's recommended to seek out vitamin B12 in the form of methylcobalamin, which is more easily absorbed.

Omega-3 from Plant Sources: Although fish oil is the most common source of omega-3 (EPA and DHA), vegans can opt for algae oil, a plant-based source that provides omega-3 in similar forms.

Vegan Vitamin D: Vitamin D3, which is more effective than D2, is often derived from lanolin (sheep's wool). However, there are vegan D3 options derived from algae.

Plant-Based Protein Powder: For those looking to increase their protein intake without animal products, there are high-quality plant-based protein powders made from peas, brown rice, hemp, and other plant sources.

Iron and Calcium: Although these minerals are available in plant sources, their absorption is sometimes lower than in animal sources. To improve absorption, it's recommended to take iron with vitamin C and avoid taking calcium and iron together, as they can interfere with each other's absorption.

Essential Supplements for Health and Performance

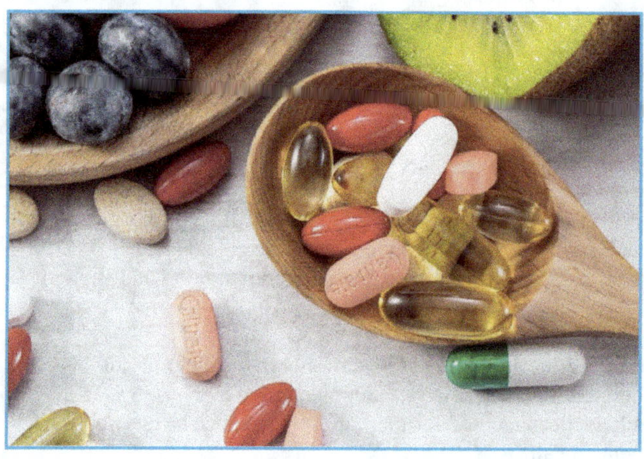

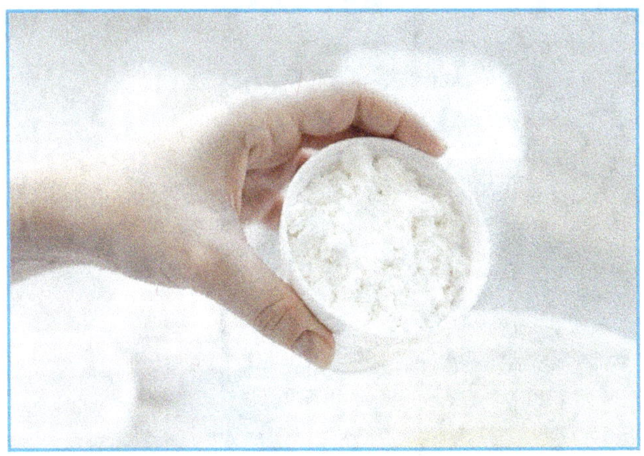

What it is and How it Works in the Body

Protein is an essential macronutrient composed of amino acids, which are the "building blocks" the body uses to develop and repair tissues. Protein is fundamental not only for muscle development and post-exercise recovery but also for the production of hormones, enzymes, and neurotransmitters. Adequate protein intake supports muscle growth, tissue synthesis, and reduces muscle breakdown.

Sources of Protein and Their Benefits

Animal Sources: Animal proteins (chicken, turkey, eggs, fish, red meat) are "complete proteins" because they contain all nine essential amino acids the body cannot produce on its own.

Plant Sources: While many plant proteins (legumes, nuts, seeds, tofu) may lack some essential amino acids, combining them strategically (such as rice and beans) can provide a complete amino acid profile.Tabla de alimentos ricos en proteínas:

Note: Supplementation is NOT a substitute for food.

Food	Source	Protein (g/100g)
Chicken	Animal	27
Turkey	Animal	29
Beef	Animal	24
Pork	Animal	27
Ham	Animal	27

Rabbit	Animal	20
Tuna	Animal	23
Hake	Animal	17
Salmon	Animal	19,3
Prawns	Animal	16
Egg (Whole)	Animal	6 Talla L
Egg White	Animal	4
Milk	Animal	3,3
Natural Yogurt	Animal	5
Cottage Cheese	Animal	11
Kefir	Animal	3,4
Lentils	Plant	25
Chickpeas	Plant	19
Green Beans	Plant	1,8
White Beans / Navy Beans	Plant	21,4
Peas	Plant	8
Almonds	Plant	21
Peanuts	Plant	24
Chia seeds	Plant	15
Pumpkin Seeds	Plant	19
Quinoa	Plant	14
Tofu	Plant	13
Edamame	Plant	11
Amaranth	Plant	13
Spelt	Plant	15
Oats	Plant	14
Pea Protein (Powder)	Plant	75
Brown Rice Protein (Powder)	Plant	70
Soy Protein (Powder)	Plant	80
Whey Protein (Powder)	Animal	80

Recommended Dosages by Goal

Maintenance: 0.8–1.2 grams per kilogram of body weight.

Muscle Gain: 1.6–2.2 grams per kilogram of body weight, divided into several intakes throughout the day to maximize muscle protein synthesis.

Recipes for This Stage:

Protein Shake:

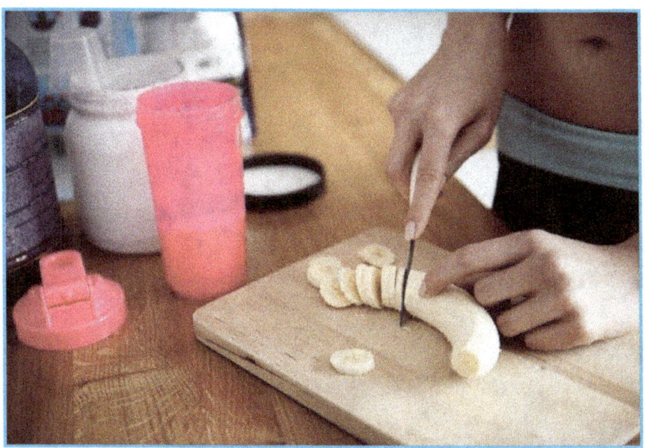

Ingredients:

- 1 cup (240 ml) milk (can use dairy, almond, soy, etc.)
- 1 medium banana (about 120 g)
- 1 tbsp (16 g) peanut butter
- 1 scoop (30 g) protein powder (any flavor)
- 1 tsp (5 g) honey (optional, for sweetness)
- ½ cup (120 ml) water or ice (optional, to adjust consistency)

Instructions:

1. Place all ingredients in a blender.

2. Blend until smooth and creamy.

3. Adjust with water or ice for desired consistency.

4. Serve and enjoy.

- Calories: 350 kcal
- Protein: 30 g
- Fat: 12 g
- Carbohydrates: 35 g

Protein Banana Bread:

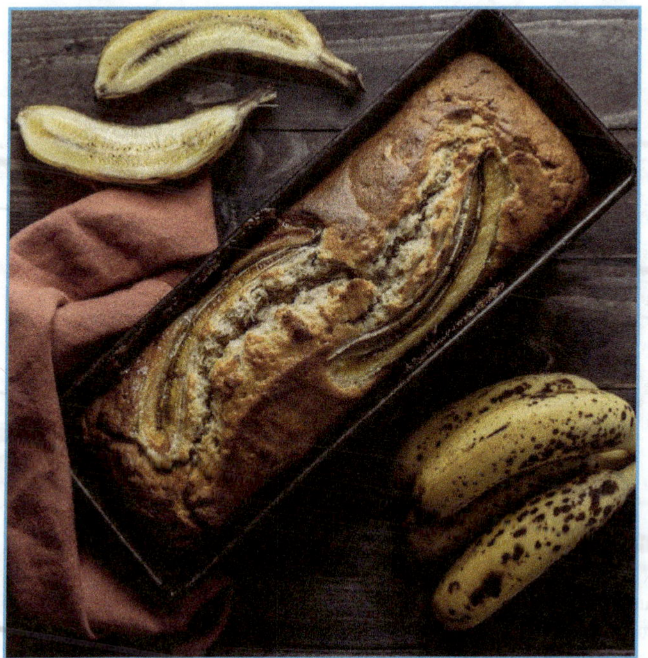

Ingredients:

- 3 ripe bananas (about 360 g)
- 2 large eggs
- 1 cup (240 ml) milk (dairy or plant-based)
- ½ cup (128 g) peanut butter
- 1 cup (120 g) oat flour (can be made by blending oats)
- 1 scoop (30 g) vanilla or banana protein powder
- 1 tsp baking soda
- 1 tsp baking powder
- ½ tsp cinnamon
- ¼ tsp salt
- 1 tsp vanilla extract

1. Preheat oven to 180°C (350°F) and grease a loaf pan.

2. In a large bowl, mash the bananas into a puree.

3. Add eggs, milk, peanut butter, and vanilla extract. Mix well.

4. In a separate bowl, combine oat flour, protein powder, baking soda, baking powder, cinnamon, and salt.

5. Gradually add the dry ingredients to the wet ingredients and mix until well combined.

6. Pour the batter into the loaf pan and bake for 45–50 minutes, or until a toothpick inserted in the center comes out clean.

7. Allow to cool before removing from the pan and slicing.

Approximate Nutritional Information (per serving, based on 10 servings):

- Calories: 200 kcal
- Protein: 10 g
- Fat: 8 g
- Carbohydrates: 25 g

For Weight Loss:

Increasing protein intake to 1.5–2 grams per kilogram helps preserve muscle mass during calorie-restricted diets.

Vegan and Plant-Based Options

Protein powders from pea, soy, brown rice, or hemp are ideal for vegans. Grains like quinoa and amaranth are also good sources of complete protein for those seeking natural alternatives.

Tips for Optimizing Absorption and Timing

Consuming protein every 3–4 hours can optimize protein synthesis. Additionally, studies show that consuming protein after exercise (within the first 30–60 minutes) is ideal for maximizing recovery and muscle growth.

Possible Side Effects and Contraindications

Excessive protein intake may impact kidney function in individuals with pre-existing kidney disease. Additionally, protein powders may cause digestive issues or allergies if they contain undesirable or low-quality ingredients.

Caffeine

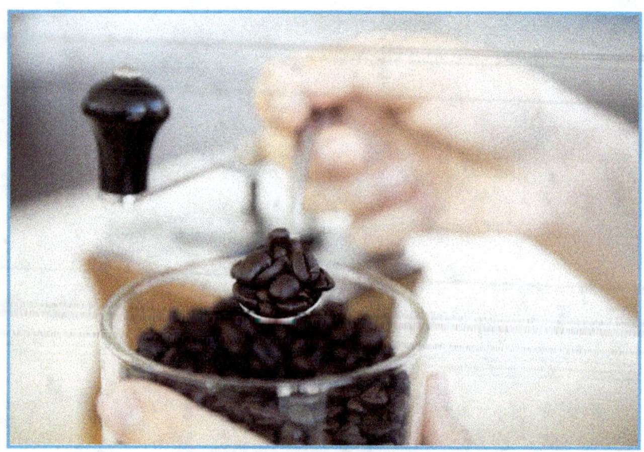

Mechanism of Action and Effects on Performance

Caffeine acts as a stimulant by blocking adenosine receptors in the brain, which reduces the sensation of fatigue and increases mental and physical alertness. It is highly effective for improving endurance, concentration, and performance in high-intensity exercises.

Benefits and Precautions of Caffeine Use

Caffeine enhances endurance and reaction time, and reduces the perceived effort during exercise. However, excessive use can lead to nervousness, anxiety, insomnia, and dependence. It is essential to start with moderate doses to assess individual tolerance.

Recommended Dosage and Timing

A dose of 3–6 mg per kilogram of body weight taken one hour before exercise is ideal for enhancing performance without excessive side effects. It is recommended to avoid caffeine late in the day, as its half-life can interfere with sleep.

Caffeine and Exercise: What Studies Say

Caffeine has been shown to improve performance in endurance sports and high-intensity exercises. Studies confirm that it enhances endurance in athletes and is one of the most effective ergogenic aids for long-duration activities.

Caffeine-Free Alternatives and Plant-Based Options

For those seeking caffeine-free options, green tea contains L-theanine, an amino acid that promotes mental calmness without caffeine's stimulation. Other options include herbs like rhodiola, which can naturally boost energy.

Creatine

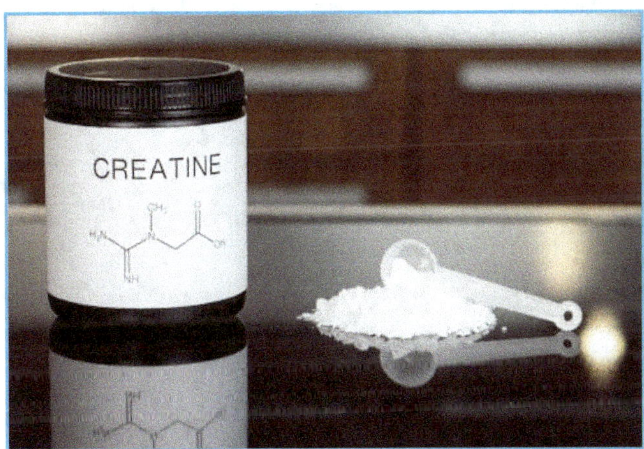

Creatine as a Key Supplement for Strength and Performance

Creatine is a naturally occurring compound in muscles that aids in the production of ATP, the primary energy source used by muscles during high-intensity, short-duration exercises.

After a few weeks of use, users often notice fuller muscles due to creatine's ability to draw water into muscle cells.

Mechanism of Action and Benefits

Creatine enhances the muscles' ability to produce energy during intense exercises, allowing for more repetitions or heavier lifting. It also supports recovery and promotes water retention in muscle cells, contributing to muscle growth.

Dosage, Types of Creatine, and How to Choose the Best Option

Dosage: A loading phase of 20 grams per day for 5–7 days, followed by a maintenance dose of 3–5 grams per day.

Types: Creatine monohydrate is the most recommended form due to its effectiveness and bioavailability. Other forms (like creatine HCl or ethyl ester) have not shown superior results in scientific studies.

Scientific Evidence on Safety and Effectiveness

Creatine has been studied for decades and is safe at recommended doses. It enhances strength and muscle growth, and no significant adverse effects have been observed with long-term use.

Note: About 5% of the body's creatine is stored in the brain. Some studies have found that it may improve memory, alertness, mental fatigue, and, in certain cases, even aid in managing depression.

Considerations for Women, Vegans, and Older Adults

Creatine is beneficial for everyone, including women and older adults. It is particularly useful for vegans, who tend to have lower natural creatine levels in their muscles due to a lack of animal-based sources in their diet.

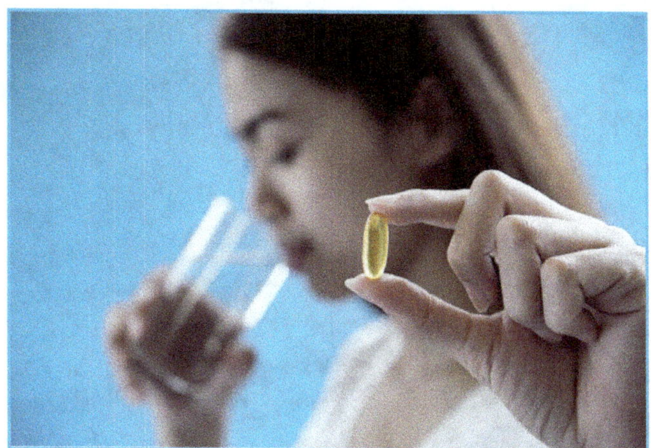

Importance of Vitamin D for the Immune System and Performance

Vitamin D is essential for calcium absorption, bone health, and proper immune function. It also plays a role in muscle function, enhancing performance and reducing the risk of injuries.

Specific Benefits for Bones, Muscles, and General Health

Vitamin D strengthens bones by aiding calcium absorption; a deficiency can lead to muscle weakness and fatigue. It's especially important for older adults to reduce the risk of falls and fractures.

Dosage Based on Levels and Sun Exposure

The recommended dose varies, but most adults can benefit from 1,000–4,000 IU daily, especially in winter or in areas with limited sun exposure.

When and How to Supplement (Seasonal Needs, Deficiencies)

Supplementation is recommended in winter months or when sun exposure is low. Taking it with meals containing fat improves absorption.

Vegan Alternatives and Food Sources

Vegan D3 derived from algae is an excellent option. UV-exposed mushrooms also provide a natural source of D2.

Magnesium

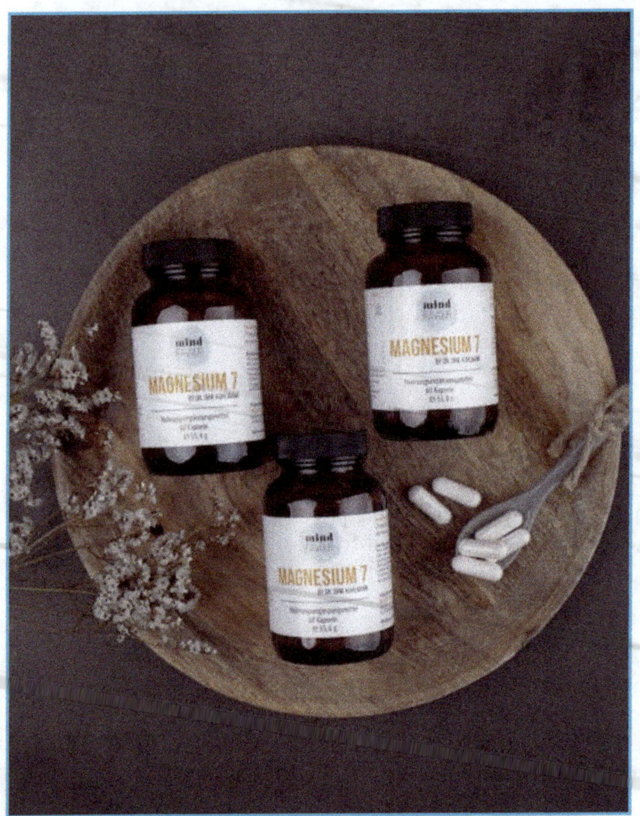

Role of Magnesium in Performance, Sleep, and Recovery

Magnesium is essential for key bodily functions, including muscle contraction, sleep, and protein synthesis. It reduces stress and improves sleep quality, aiding in post-exercise recovery.

Recommended Dosage and Types of Magnesium

A daily intake of 300–400 mg is recommended. Different forms offer varying bioavailability: magnesium citrate is more easily absorbed, while magnesium oxide is less effective but more economical.

Is Supplementation Necessary? Groups at Risk of Deficiency

People under stress, athletes, and those with diets low in magnesium may benefit from supplementation. A magnesium deficiency can lead to cramps, fatigue, and sleep issues.

Tips to Maximize Absorption (Useful Combinations)

Taking magnesium with calcium and vitamin D enhances absorption. Consuming it at night promotes sleep and relaxation.

Side Effects and Precautions

Excessive magnesium can cause diarrhea and stomach discomfort. People with kidney problems should consult a doctor before supplementing.

Vitamin B12

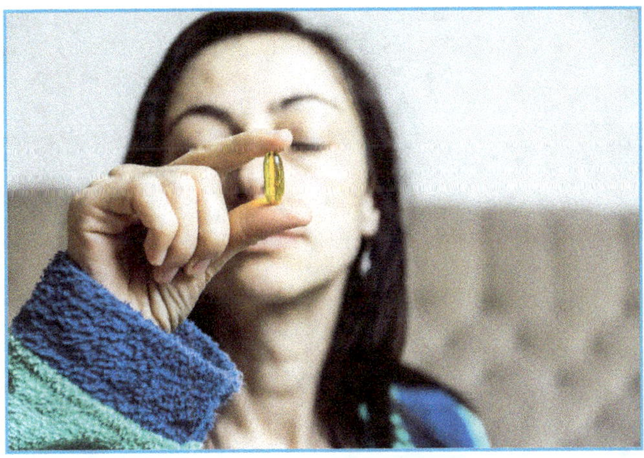

Fundamental Role of Vitamin B12 in Energy and Metabolism

B12 is crucial for energy metabolism, red blood cell production, and nervous system function. A deficiency can lead to fatigue, anemia, and neurological issues.

Dosage and Recommendations for Vegans and Vegetarians

For vegans, a dose of 250 mcg daily or 1,000 mcg twice a week is recommended.

How to Detect Deficiencies and When to Supplement

A blood test can reveal low levels. Symptoms of deficiency include fatigue, muscle weakness, and mental fog.

Vegetarian Sources and Practical Recommendations

Fortified foods and supplements in the form of cyanocobalamin or methylcobalamin are safe and effective options.

Consequences of Deficiency and Supplementation Safety

Untreated B12 deficiency can cause permanent neurological damage. Supplementation is safe as excess B12 is eliminated through the kidneys.

Omega-3

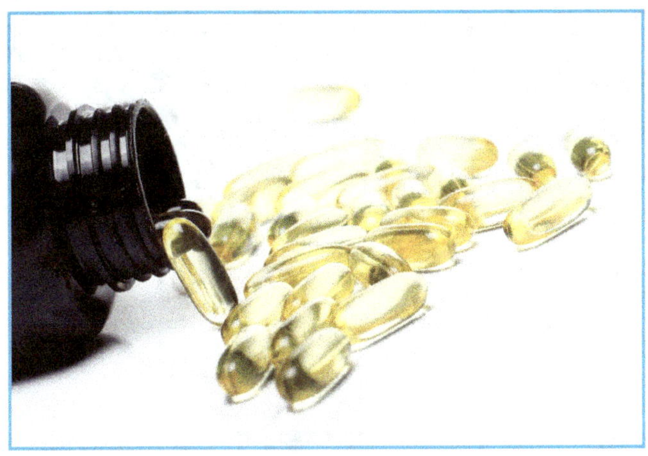

Effects of Omega-3 on Brain, Heart, and Muscle Recovery

Omega-3s are essential for cardiovascular health, brain function, and inflammation reduction, benefiting muscle recovery.

Recommended Dosage and Primary Sources (Animal and Plant-Based)

250–500 mg of EPA and DHA daily. Sources include fish oil and, for vegans, algae oil.

Comparison of Fish Oil, Algae, and Other Plant Oils

Algae oil is a plant-based equivalent to fish oil, providing EPA and DHA in similar amounts.

Scientific Evidence and Recent Studies

Omega 3s are scientifically supported for reducing cardiovascular disease risk and improving cognitive function and post-exercise recovery.

Ideal Supplementation for Vegans and Practical Options

Algae oil is the best vegan option, rich in EPA and DHA.

Benefits of CoQ10 in Energy and Cardiovascular Health

Coenzyme Q10 (CoQ10) is a natural antioxidant essential for cellular energy production. CoQ10 is especially important for high-energy organs like the heart and muscles. It primarily functions in the electron transport chain in mitochondria, the cell's "powerhouses," and is also a potent antioxidant that protects against cellular damage.

Mechanism of Action and Optimal Dosage

CoQ10 aids ATP production and reduces oxidative stress, supporting cardiovascular health and reducing muscle fatigue. Recommended doses range from 90 to 200 mg daily, but some individuals may require up to 300 mg depending on levels and specific goals.

Who Should Consider Supplementation?

Older Adults: Natural CoQ10 production decreases with age, so older adults may benefit from supplementation.

People with Heart Disease or Hypertension: CoQ10 is beneficial for improving heart function in those with heart failure, high blood pressure, or cardiovascular diseases.

People with Chronic Fatigue or Endurance Athletes: Given its role in energy production, CoQ10 is useful for those needing improved endurance and reduced muscle fatigue.

Interactions and Precautions with Other Supplements or Medications

CoQ10 can interact with certain medications, especially anticoagulants like warfarin, reducing their effectiveness. It's also advisable to consult a professional before combining it with supplements like vitamin K or other antioxidants.

Vegan Sources and Key Scientific Data

CoQ10 is found in small amounts in foods like fish, meat, and nuts, but these typically do not provide therapeutic doses. For vegans, CoQ10 supplements derived from bacterial fermentation are a suitable alternative. CoQ10 is widely studied, with evidence supporting its effectiveness in cardiovascular support and muscle fatigue reduction.

Melatonin

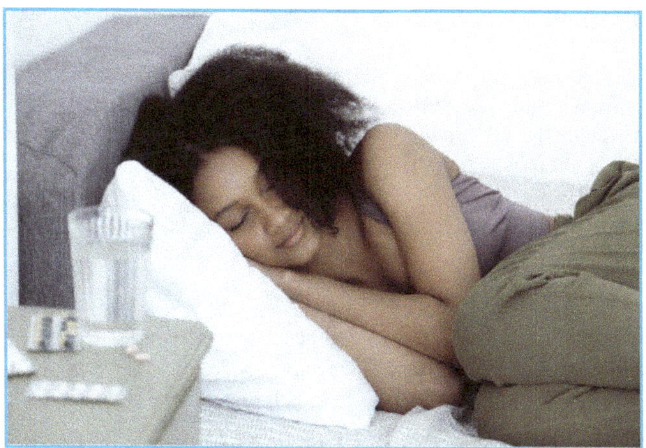

Melatonin and Its Role in Sleep Regulation

Melatonin is a natural hormone produced by the pineal gland in the brain, responsible for regulating the sleep-wake cycle. Melatonin production increases in the dark, helping the body prepare for sleep, and decreases during the day, promoting wakefulness.

Dosage, Timing, and Potential Side Effects

Melatonin is commonly used as a supplement to improve sleep quality and treat jet lag. The ideal dose depends on the person and goal:

For Insomnia: 1–5 mg about 30–60 minutes before bed is recommended.

For Jet Lag: 0.5–3 mg before bedtime on the first day of travel, continuing for a few days to adjust sleep.

Generally, melatonin is safe, though some people may experience mild side effects like daytime drowsiness, dizziness, or headaches if the dose is too high.

Recommendations for Jet Lag and Sleep Disturbances

Melatonin is helpful for frequent travelers experiencing jet lag, as it helps adapt the sleep cycle to a new schedule. It can also be beneficial for night-shift workers or people with irregular sleep schedules. For those with chronic sleep issues, starting with the minimum effective dose is recommended.

Natural Alternatives and Precautions

Foods like cherries, walnuts, and oats naturally contain small amounts of melatonin. Other alternatives include valerian and passionflower, which also promote sleep and relaxation. Long-term melatonin use is not recommended without consulting a professional, as prolonged use could reduce natural melatonin production in the body.

Scientific Evidence and Its Relation to Sleep Quality

Melatonin is one of the most studied sleep supplements and has proven effective in improving sleep onset and quality. Studies indicate it is especially beneficial for people with circadian rhythm disruptions due to travel or shift work, helping reduce fatigue and improve cognitive function.

Ashwagandha

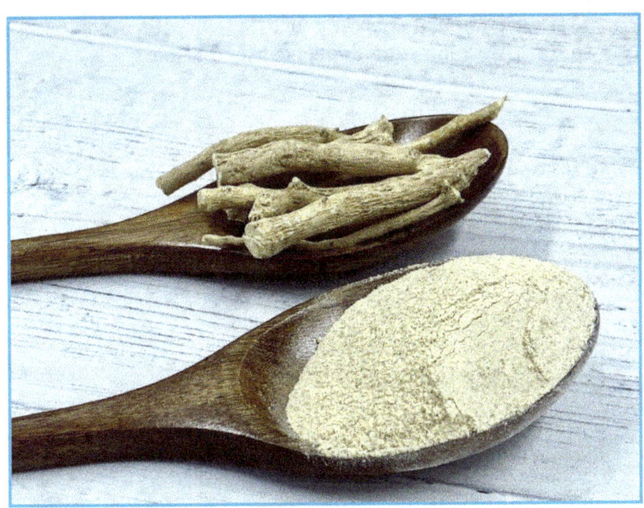

Natural Adaptogen and Its Effects on Stress and Energy

Ashwagandha is an adaptogenic herb used in Ayurvedic medicine, popular for its ability to reduce stress, improve mood, and boost energy levels. Adaptogens help the body manage stress by regulating cortisol, the primary stress hormone.

Recommended Dosage and Proven Benefits

The recommended dosage ranges from 300 to 600 mg daily of standardized ashwagandha root extract, which is the most studied form. Ashwagandha's benefits include:

Stress Reduction: Studies have shown that ashwagandha reduces cortisol levels, alleviating symptoms of anxiety and stress.

Cognitive Function and Mood Improvement: Research suggests it can enhance memory, concentration, and mood, making it beneficial for mental well-being.

Increased Energy and Physical Performance: In a fitness context, ashwagandha has been found to improve muscle strength, endurance, and post-exercise recovery.

Side Effects and Contraindications

Ashwagandha is generally safe for most people, though some may experience mild side effects such as stomach discomfort or drowsiness. Caution is advised for individuals with autoimmune disorders, as it may stimulate the immune system. It's also not recommended during pregnancy or breastfeeding without medical supervision.

Vegan Ashwagandha Alternatives and Options for Natural Consumers

Ashwagandha powder or capsules are typically vegan. For those preferring alternatives, other adaptogens like rhodiola and ginseng also reduce stress and improve energy without stimulating the immune system.

Research on Exercise and Recovery

Research shows that ashwagandha not only helps reduce stress but also improves muscle strength and endurance in athletes. In an eight-week study, participants taking ashwagandha experienced significant gains in muscle mass and strength, making it an excellent choice for those looking to boost both physical and mental performance.

Practical Supplementation Guide by Personal Needs

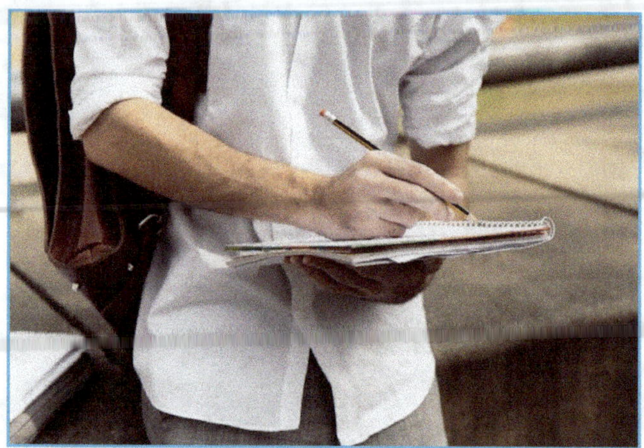

Supplementation can be a powerful tool when tailored to each person's unique needs, goals, and lifestyle. This guide is designed to help you customize your supplementation plan safely and effectively. Whether you aim to improve physical performance, support mental health, promote longevity, or simply cover basic needs, aligning supplements with your specific goals will maximize benefits and avoid unnecessary use.

Personalization is key to making supplementation have a positive impact on your life. Here's a step-by-step guide to designing your supplementation plan:

Define Your Specific Goals: Ask yourself about your main priorities. Do you want to build muscle and improve performance? Is your focus on reducing stress and improving sleep? Or are you interested in promoting longevity and general health? Having clear goals will help you select supplements that truly make a difference.

Evaluate Your Current Diet and Lifestyle: The foundation of any supplementation plan is a balanced diet. Analyze your nutrient intake to identify deficiencies or areas that could benefit from reinforcement. For example, if you follow a vegan diet, you may need vitamin B12 and plant-based omega-3 supplements.

Consider Your Individual Characteristics: Factors like age, gender, physical activity level, health status, and stress levels influence your supplementation needs. Older adults may benefit from vitamin D and calcium for bone health, while growing teenagers may need additional protein and iron.

Consult a Professional: While many supplements are safe, it's advisable to consult a professional, especially if you have pre-existing health conditions, take medications, or are unsure about the appropriate doses for your needs.

Review Scientific Evidence: Choose supplements backed by research with proven effects. Supplementation research has advanced significantly, so selecting products with solid evidence and, preferably, from certified brands, will help you avoid ineffective or risky supplements.

Listen to Your Body and Adjust as Needed: Once you start taking a supplement, observe how your body responds. If you notice improvements in energy, performance, or overall well-being, it's a good sign. Conversely, if you experience side effects or no changes, it may indicate that the supplement isn't right for you or that the dose needs adjustment.

Supplements by Goals: Performance, Mental Health, and Longevity

Each health and wellness goal has specific requirements, and supplements can play different roles depending on the focus. Below are recommendations for key supplements aligned with various goals.

1. Physical Performance

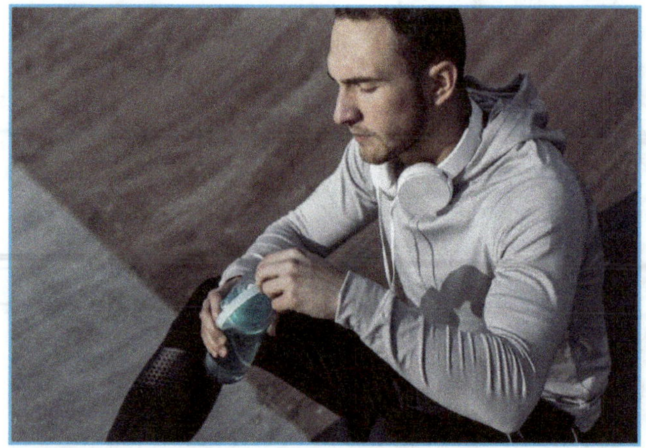

Supplements for physical performance aim to improve strength, endurance, recovery, and muscle growth.

Protein: Essential for muscle protein synthesis and post-workout recovery.

Recommended Dose: 1.6–2.2 grams per kilogram of body weight, divided across several meals daily.

Creatine: Enhances strength and power in high-intensity exercises and supports muscle gain.

Recommended Dose: Loading phase of 20 grams daily for 5–7 days, followed by a maintenance dose of 3–5 grams daily.

Beta-Alanine: Reduces muscle fatigue in high-intensity exercises and improves endurance.

Recommended Dose: 3–6 grams daily, divided into 1–2 gram doses.

Caffeine: Increases alertness and reduces perceived effort, useful for endurance sports and general performance.

Recommended Dose: 3–6 mg per kilogram of body weight, taken 30–60 minutes before training.

2. Mental Health

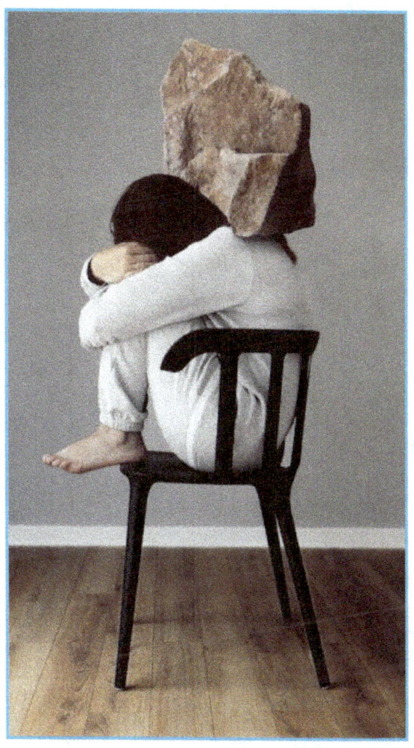

Supplements for mental health focus on reducing stress, improving sleep, and supporting mental clarity and concentration.

Magnesium: Contributes to muscle relaxation and helps regulate cortisol, the stress hormone.

Recommended Dose: 300–400 mg daily, ideally before bedtime.

Ashwagandha: An adaptogen known for reducing stress and anxiety, and improving focus.

Recommended Dose: 300–600 mg daily of standardized extract.

Omega-3 (EPA and DHA): Enhances brain function and reduces inflammation.

Recommended Dose: 250–500 mg of combined EPA and DHA daily.

Melatonin: Ideal for those needing to regulate sleep cycles, melatonin improves sleep quality.

Recommended Dose: 0.5–5 mg before bed, depending on sensitivity and individual need.

3. Longevity and General Well-being

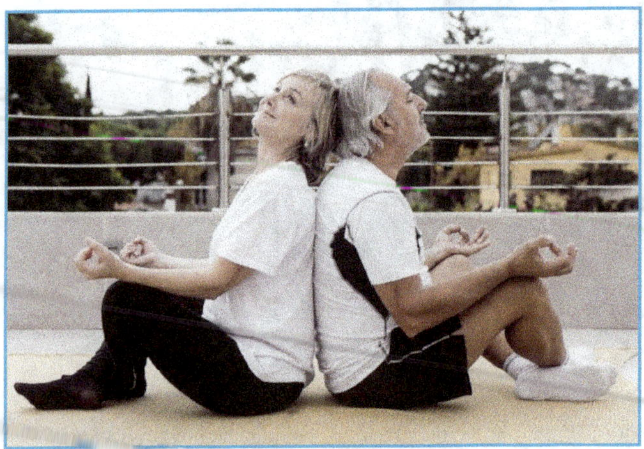

Supplements for longevity and general well-being support long-term health, prevent disease, and help maintain an active and healthy life.

Vitamin D: Essential for bone health, immune function, and muscle function.

Recommended Dose: 1,000–4,000 IU daily, adjusted according to sun exposure and blood tests.

Coenzyme Q10: An antioxidant supporting cardiovascular health and cellular energy, particularly important for older adults.

Recommended Dose: 90–200 mg daily, preferably with a fat-containing meal.

Vitamin B12: Necessary for energy production and brain function, especially important for vegans and older adults.

Recommended Dose: 250 mcg daily or 1,000 mcg twice a week.

Curcumin: A natural antioxidant and anti-inflammatory beneficial for joint health and general wellness.

Recommended Dose: 500–1,000 mg daily of curcumin extract with piperine to improve absorption.

Recommendations for Adolescents, Adults, and Older Adults

Your life stage directly impacts your nutritional and supplementation needs. Here are specific recommendations for each age group:

Adolescents

Adolescence is a period of rapid growth and development. While a balanced diet is the foundation, some supplements may be helpful:

Protein: For active teens or those involved in sports, 1.2–1.5 grams of protein per kilogram of body weight can aid recovery and muscle growth.

Iron: Particularly important for teenage girls, as iron needs increase with the onset of menstruation. Deficiency can lead to fatigue and reduced performance.

Omega-3: Beneficial for brain development and academic performance.

Recommended Dose: 250–500 mg of EPA and DHA daily.

Note: Supplementation for teenagers should be monitored and preferably guided by a healthcare professional.

Adults

Adults can benefit from supplementation that supports both physical performance and general health:

High-Quality Multivitamin: Covers potential deficiencies in essential nutrients, especially for those with restrictive diets or demanding lifestyles.

Vitamin D and Magnesium: Vitamin D is crucial for bone health, while magnesium aids in stress management and sleep quality.

Protein and Creatine: Beneficial for physically active adults looking to enhance performance and recovery.

Older Adults

In older adults, supplementation can help maintain bone health, prevent disease, and preserve cognitive function:

Calcium and Vitamin D: Essential for preventing osteoporosis and strengthening bones.

Recommended Dose: 1,000–4,000 IU of vitamin D daily, and 1,000–1,200 mg of calcium daily.

Coenzyme Q10 and Omega-3: Support cardiovascular health, brain function, and boost energy and vitality.

Vitamin B12: Older adults have reduced B12 absorption, so supplementing is crucial to prevent deficiencies.

Recommended Dose: 250–500 mcg daily.

Quick Reference Table by Supplement Type and Dosage

A quick reference table is included below for easy access to recommended dosages and specific targets for each supplement:

Supplement	Goal	Recommended Dose
Protein	Maintenance, Muscle Gain	1.2–2.2 g/kg of body weight
Creatine	Strength, Power	3–5 g daily (loading phase: 20 g/day)
Magnesium	Relaxation, Sleep	300–400 mg daily
Omega-3	Brain, Heart Health	250–500 mg EPA and DHA
Vitamin D	Bone, Immune Health	1,000–4,000 IU daily
Vitamin B12	Energy, Brain Function	250–500 mcg daily
Melatonin	Sleep	0.5–5 mg before bed
Ashwagandha	Stress Reduction, Energy	300–600 mg daily

Tips to Boost Supplementation Effects

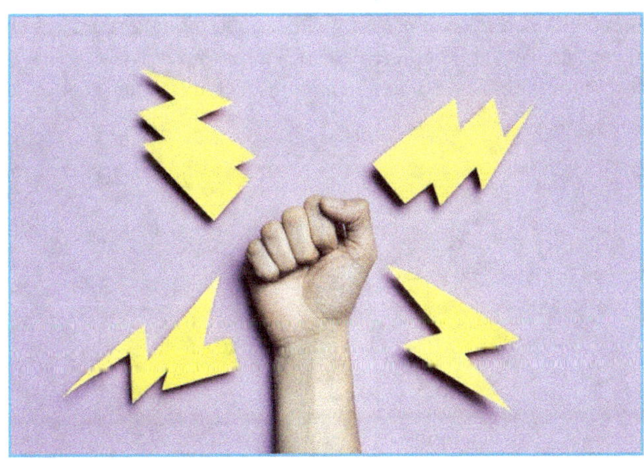

Supplementation is just one piece of the health and performance puzzle. To achieve the best results, it's crucial to integrate supplements within a lifestyle that balances diet, exercise, and rest. Additionally, understanding supplement combinations that enhance each other's effects, following circadian rhythms, and adopting optimal habits can make a significant difference in the benefits you experience. This chapter provides strategies to maximize the effects of your supplements and reach your goals more effectively.

The Relationship Between Exercise, Diet, and Rest

Exercise

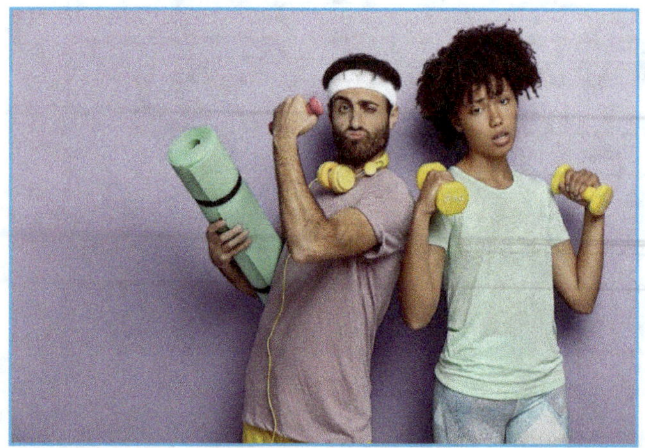

Physical activity is essential for maximizing performance-oriented supplementation, as training stimulates muscle growth, cardiovascular endurance, and metabolic function. Combining specific supplements (like creatine or protein) with a good training routine enables the body to utilize these nutrients more efficiently. Additionally, recovery supplements (such as magnesium or amino acids) help repair muscle damage and reduce fatigue after exercise.

Practical Tip: Plan your workout to maximize supplement effects. For example, if you take caffeine before training, use it on intense or high-endurance days to benefit from its energy and focus effects.

Diet

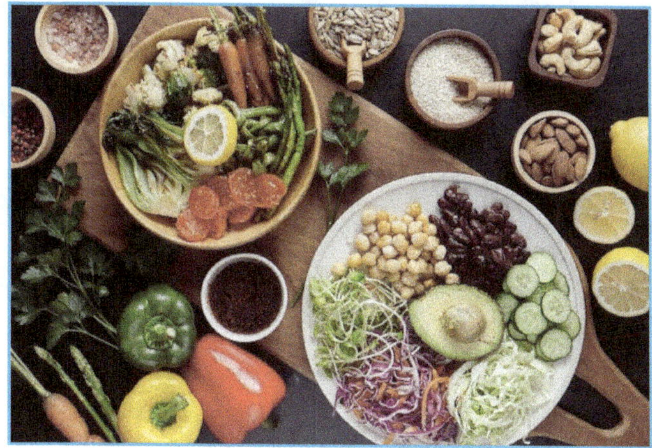

Diet is the foundation of any supplementation program. No supplement can replace an unbalanced diet. Nutrients from food are the primary source of energy and wellness; supplementation should support, not replace, these nutrients. Additionally, some supplements are more effective when taken with food. For example, vitamin D and CoQ10 are better absorbed with a meal rich in healthy fats.

Practical Tip: Ensure a balanced diet with sufficient protein, carbohydrates, and healthy fats to make your supplementation effective. Include foods rich in fiber, vitamins, and minerals to optimize overall health.

Rest

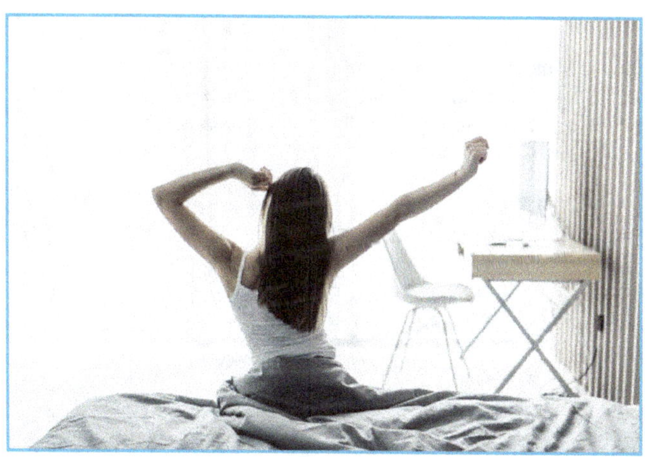

Rest and recovery are essential for both physical and mental performance. During sleep, the body repairs muscle tissue, regulates hormones like testosterone and cortisol, and consolidates memory and learning. Supplements like melatonin, magnesium, and ashwagandha can help improve sleep quality and promote relaxation, allowing the body to restore energy levels and be ready for the next day's training.

Practical Tip: Create a regular sleep routine, and if needed, consider supplementing with melatonin or magnesium to improve sleep quality. Remember, deep and adequate rest enhances the effects of any supplement, as the body is in an optimal state to absorb nutrients.

Useful Combinations and Synergistic Supplements

Certain supplement combinations enhance each other's effects, improving absorption or effectiveness in the body. Here are some of the most useful synergistic combinations:

Protein + Creatine

Protein and creatine are a classic combination for muscle gain and performance. Protein provides the amino acids needed for muscle synthesis, while creatine supplies energy for high-intensity training. Taking them together post-workout helps improve recovery and muscle growth.

Vitamin D + Calcium

Vitamin D improves calcium absorption in the intestine, strengthening bones and reducing fracture risk, especially in older adults. This combination is ideal for those looking to prevent bone issues and strengthen the musculoskeletal system.

Omega-3 + Antioxidants (like Vitamin E)

Omega-3s have anti-inflammatory properties that benefit cardiovascular and mental health. Combined with antioxidants like vitamin E, they reduce oxidative stress, protect cells, and improve muscle recovery.

Magnesium + Vitamin B6

Magnesium and vitamin B6 work together to reduce stress, improve sleep, and support the nervous system. This combination is helpful for those seeking better relaxation and sleep quality, as well as improved muscle function.

Caffeine + L-Theanine

Caffeine boosts energy and alertness, but it may also cause anxiety or jitters in some people. L-theanine, an amino acid found in green tea, promotes relaxation without sedation. Combined, they create a state of calm alertness, ideal for enhancing focus and cognitive performance without caffeine overstimulation.

Circadian Rhythms and the Best Time for Each Supplement

Circadian rhythms are the body's natural 24-hour cycles that regulate physiological functions, including sleep, metabolism, and hormone levels. Taking supplements at the right time according to these rhythms can optimize their effectiveness.

Morning Supplements

Vitamin D: Since this vitamin is synthesized from sunlight, it's ideal to take it in the morning to align with the body's natural rhythms.

Caffeine: If you use caffeine for performance, consume it in the morning or before training. Avoid it in the afternoon or evening, as it can interfere with sleep.

B-Complex Vitamins: B vitamins help convert food into energy, so taking them in the morning optimizes energy levels throughout the day.

Midday or Post-Workout Supplements

Protein and Creatine: These supplements are ideal post-workout to improve recovery and support muscle growth.

Omega-3: Taking omega-3 with a meal rich in healthy fats enhances absorption. Taking it at midday helps maintain anti-inflammatory effects and a sense of well-being throughout the afternoon.

Evening Supplements

Magnesium: Taking magnesium at night helps relax the body and prepares it for quality sleep.

Melatonin: Taking it 30–60 minutes before bedtime helps regulate sleep, especially for those with difficulty falling asleep.

Ashwagandha: This adaptogen can be taken at night to reduce stress and anxiety and promote relaxation. It also helps lower cortisol levels, which supports better rest.

Practical Tip: Consider the time of day and your natural rhythms when planning your supplementation. This will help you align the benefits of the supplements with the specific needs of each part of the day.

Habits to Optimize Physical and Mental Performance

In addition to supplementation, adopting healthy habits boosts physical and mental performance. These habits maximize supplement effects and help maintain optimal health:

Stay Adequately Hydrated

Dehydration impacts concentration, physical performance, and recovery capacity. Drinking enough water and electrolytes throughout the day improves nutrient absorption and the effectiveness of many supplements, especially those that aid physical performance, like creatine.

Optimize Nutrition with Nutrient-Rich Foods

While supplements can fill some gaps, it's ideal to obtain most nutrients through a varied, balanced diet. Foods rich in vitamins, minerals, and antioxidants provide a solid foundation that complements the benefits of supplementation.

Establish a Consistent Sleep Routine

Lack of sleep negatively affects recovery, mental performance, and hormonal balance. Establishing a regular routine, along with supplements like magnesium or melatonin if needed, helps optimize rest and readiness for training.

Practice Breathing Exercises and Relaxation Techniques

Chronic stress interferes with the absorption and effectiveness of certain supplements, especially those aimed at improving mental health and performance. Incorporating breathing and relaxation techniques, such as meditation or yoga, helps reduce stress and increases the body's ability to benefit from supplementation.

Regularly Evaluate and Adjust Your Supplementation

Your body's needs change over time and with goals. Periodically review your supplementation plan, observe how you feel, and make adjustments based on changes in activity, diet, or health. This approach avoids over-reliance on supplements and optimizes their use mindfully.

Strategies for Motivation and Mindset to Achieve Your Goals

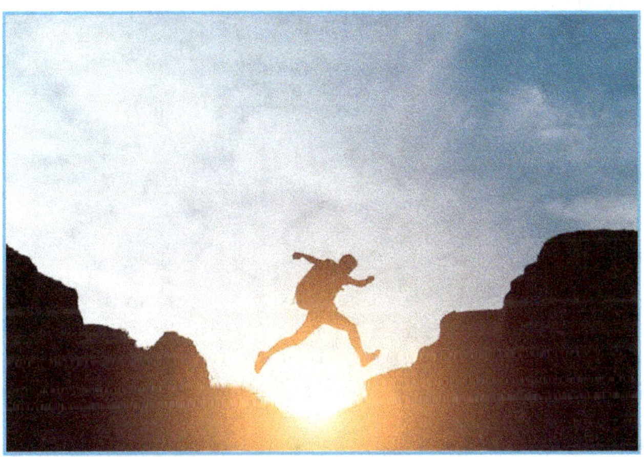

Mindset is as important as nutrition, exercise, and supplementation when it comes to reaching your health and wellness goals. Cultivating a positive attitude and building motivational and resilient skills are essential for staying on track, especially when challenges arise. This chapter will help you understand how a strong mindset and sustained motivation can transform your goals into results.

The Importance of a Positive Mindset

Your mindset largely determines how you handle challenges, interpret success, and respond to setbacks. The way you think directly impacts your habits and your ability to sustain prolonged effort. Here are some key points on how a positive mindset influences your progress:

Develop Self-Compassion and Patience: It's common to be self-critical when you don't reach a goal or experience a setback. A positive mindset, however, involves practicing self-compassion, understanding that change is gradual, and recognizing that every step, even small ones, contribute to progress.

Shift Focus to the Process, Not Just the Outcome: Focusing solely on the end result, like "losing 5 kg" or "increasing my strength by 20%," can lead to frustration if progress is slow. Instead, focus on the process—consistent training and daily dietary improvements—creating a sense of satisfaction and ongoing motivation.

Impact on Body and Health: A positive mindset reduces stress, improves recovery, and strengthens the immune system. Studies show that an optimistic attitude can boost physical performance and adherence to training and nutrition plans.

Tip: Practice "positive reframing" when you encounter a challenge. For example, rather than seeing a week without progress as a "failure," view it as an opportunity to evaluate and adjust your habits. Changing your perspective will help you stay motivated over the long term.

Setting SMART Goals

To maintain motivation, you need clear, achievable goals. SMART goals are an effective way to define your objectives in a concrete and measurable way. SMART stands for:

Specific: Define exactly what you want to achieve. Avoid vague terms like "get in shape." Instead, set specific goals like "work out four times a week."

Measurable: You should be able to measure your progress. For example, "lose 3 kg in two months" or "increase my bench press by 5 kg."

Achievable: Set goals that you can realistically reach based on your current situation. If you're a beginner, don't set advanced targets right away; start with small steps and build up gradually.

Relevant: Your goals should align with your values and personal desires. Ask yourself why the goal is important to you and ensure it genuinely motivates you.

Time-bound: Set a deadline for achieving your goal. This creates a sense of urgency and allows you to review your progress within a specific timeframe.

Example of a SMART Goal: "I want to improve my endurance by running 5 km without stopping in the next three months, training at least three times a week."

Tip: Review your goals each month and adjust them if necessary. As you progress, set new goals to keep yourself motivated.

Visualization and Success Mindset

Visualization is a mindset technique that involves vividly imagining yourself achieving your goals. Visualizing success and overcoming obstacles reinforces confidence and encourages you to keep going.

Create a Clear Picture of Your Achievements: If your goal is to improve physical performance, visualize yourself completing a workout, feeling strong, energized, and satisfied. The more realistic the visualization, the more powerful its impact.

Regular Visualization Practice: Spend 5 to 10 minutes a day visualizing your goals, especially before training or during moments of discouragement. This practice activates the brain areas associated with effort and achievement, which can improve real-life performance.

Believe in Your Ability to Achieve Your Goals: Visualization is not only about imagining the end goal but also reinforcing confidence in your ability to achieve it. When you visualize reaching your goals, your brain begins to associate those goals with real potential.

Tip: Before each training session or each week, take a moment to visualize how you want to feel at the end of the process. This strengthens your intention and helps you train with purpose.

Self-Motivation Techniques

Motivation isn't always constant; there will be days when you don't feel like working out or eating well. Here are some techniques to help you stay focused and motivated:

Remember Your "Why"

Think about the main reason driving you to improve your health and fitness. Writing it down and placing it somewhere visible will remind you in moments of weakness. When you know why you're doing something, it's easier to find the motivation to do it.

Break Your Goals Into Small Milestones

Instead of focusing only on the end goal, break it down into smaller, achievable milestones. Celebrating each accomplishment—like increasing your lifting weight or completing a week of balanced eating—keeps you motivated and gives you a sense of progress.

Develop a Reward Routine

Associate your achievements with positive rewards. You could treat yourself after reaching an important milestone, like enjoying a special meal or buying new workout gear. Rewards create a motivational system that reinforces your efforts.

Use Positive Affirmations

Affirmations are statements that reinforce your intentions and confidence. Phrases like "I am consistent and capable of reaching my goals" or "Every day, I'm getting closer to my best self" can help you stay focused on your objectives.

Tip: Create a "motivation board" with photos, phrases, and written goals to visualize what you want to achieve. Place it somewhere you can see daily to remind you why the effort is worthwhile.

Overcoming Obstacles and Restructuring Thoughts

The path to any goal is filled with challenges, and resilience is key to overcoming them. Resilience is the ability to face and recover from setbacks without abandoning your goals. Here are some strategies to build this skill:

Restructure Negative Thoughts

When thoughts like "this is too hard" or "I'm not capable of doing this" arise, try to reframe them. Instead of focusing on the obstacle, shift your attention to what you can do. For example, rather than "I'm not progressing fast enough," think, "I'm doing my best and making progress every day."

See Obstacles as Growth Opportunities

Every obstacle is an opportunity to learn and improve. If you have a tough week or experience a setback, take time to understand what happened and how you can overcome it in the future. This approach strengthens your ability to keep going even when problems arise.

Practice Self-Compassion and Avoid Excessive Self-Criticism

It's common to be hard on yourself when things don't go as planned. However, excessive self-criticism reduces motivation and can lead to giving up on goals. Instead, practice self-compassion: give yourself credit for your efforts and recognize that everyone has good and bad days.

Build Resilience Day by Day

Resilience is developed gradually. You can strengthen it daily by facing small challenges and adopting a mindset of continuous learning. The key is to be consistent and to view each step as a valuable contribution to your goals.

Tip: Each time you face an obstacle, take a moment to reflect on what you learned and how you can apply that knowledge next time. This practice reinforces a growth mindset and helps you move forward despite difficulties.

Supplementation for Recovery and Injury Prevention

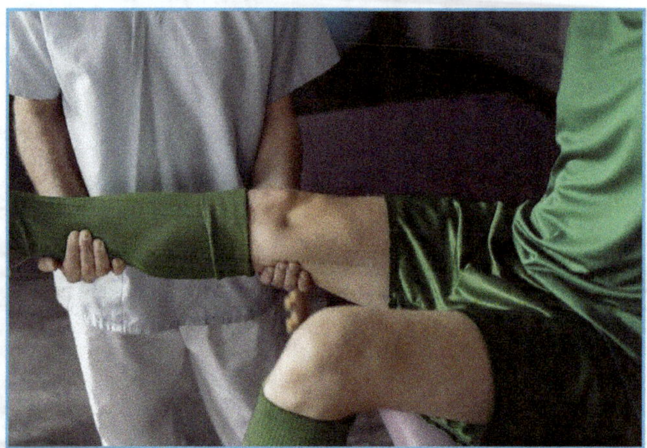

For anyone who regularly practices sports or trains consistently, recovery and injury prevention are key to maintaining performance and long-term health. This chapter explores supplements that help reduce inflammation, improve joint health, and speed up muscle recovery, along with additional strategies to optimize rest and prevent overtraining.

Natural Anti-Inflammatory Supplements: Omega-3, Turmeric, and Resveratrol

Inflammation is a natural response of the body to exercise stress, but chronic or excessive inflammation can slow recovery and increase the risk of injury. Here are some natural anti-inflammatory supplements to help reduce inflammation and improve recovery:

Omega-3 (EPA and DHA)

Omega-3 fatty acids, especially EPA and DHA, have anti-inflammatory properties that can help reduce muscle soreness and improve joint health. Found in fish oil, krill oil, and algae oil (ideal for vegans), omega-3s are also essential for cardiovascular health, which benefits overall performance and recovery.

Recommended Dose: 250–500 mg of combined EPA and DHA daily, preferably with a fat-rich meal to enhance absorption.

Turmeric (Curcumin)

Curcumin, the active compound in turmeric, is known for its anti-inflammatory and antioxidant properties. It can help reduce post-workout muscle pain and improve flexibility and mobility. Curcumin is best absorbed when taken with piperine (black pepper extract).

Recommended Dose: 500–1,000 mg of curcumin extract with piperine daily.

Resveratrol

This antioxidant, found in grape skins and red wine, has shown anti-inflammatory effects and helps protect against oxidative stress. Resveratrol also aids recovery and may reduce cell damage caused by intense training.

Recommended Dose: 200–500 mg daily.

Tip: These supplements support recovery and offer general health benefits, making them an integral part of a comprehensive approach to long-term inflammation reduction.

Joint Health Supplements: Glucosamine, Chondroitin, and Collagen

Joint health is essential for anyone training regularly, as joints are especially vulnerable to wear and tear over time. Keeping joints strong and well-nourished is key to injury prevention.

Glucosamine

Glucosamine is a natural compound that helps maintain joint cartilage. It reduces pain and stiffness and prevents further cartilage deterioration. Often used for osteoarthritis symptoms, it can benefit people who engage in high-impact sports.

Recommended Dose: 1,500 mg daily, ideally with meals for better absorption.

Chondroitin

Chondroitin complements glucosamine and helps reduce cartilage wear. It has been shown to improve cartilage elasticity and resilience, reduce joint pain, and improve mobility for those experiencing joint discomfort.

Recommended Dose: 800–1,200 mg daily, generally combined with glucosamine.

Collagen

Collagen is a structural protein vital for connective tissue, tendons, and ligaments. Supplementing with collagen can improve tissue elasticity and reduce joint pain, especially in individuals with joint wear or athletes who put heavy loads on their joints. Studies have also found collagen to benefit skin health and other tissues.

Recommended Dose: 10–15 grams of hydrolyzed collagen daily, ideally in the morning or before training.

Tip: The combination of glucosamine, chondroitin, and collagen is an effective strategy for strengthening joints and preventing wear. It is especially recommended for high-impact sports like running, CrossFit, and weightlifting.

Muscle Recovery: The Importance of BCAAs, Protein, and Magnesium in Post-Workout Recovery

Muscle recovery is essential for avoiding injuries, improving endurance, and ensuring muscle growth. Recovery-supporting supplements allow the body to better adapt to training demands.

BCAAs (Branched-Chain Amino Acids)

BCAAs, which include leucine, isoleucine, and valine, are essential amino acids directly used by muscles. They help reduce fatigue and muscle soreness and improve protein synthesis. BCAAs are particularly beneficial for those who train on an empty stomach or engage in prolonged exercise sessions.

Recommended Dose: 5–10 grams before or after training.

Protein

Protein is essential for recovery, muscle growth, and tissue repair. Adequate daily protein intake helps maintain muscle mass and reduces the risk of injury due to overtraining. Protein powders, such as whey or plant-based proteins, are ideal for those who need a protein boost after training.

Recommended Dose: 1.6–2.2 grams of protein per kilogram of body weight daily, spread across meals.

Magnesium

Magnesium is essential for muscle and nerve function and helps reduce cramps and post-workout soreness. It also improves muscle relaxation and sleep, which promotes better recovery. Taking it at night is ideal to optimize its relaxing effect.

Recommended Dose: 300–400 mg daily, preferably in the evening to improve sleep and recovery.

Tip: BCAAs are ideal for quick recovery after intense exercise, while protein and magnesium support overall recovery and help maintain long-term muscle mass.

Additional Recovery Strategies

In addition to supplementation, there are complementary practices that help reduce injury risk and improve muscle recovery:

Massage and Compression Therapy

Massages help reduce muscle tension, improve circulation, and reduce the risk of muscle knots. Compression therapy, such as compression socks or pressure devices, can speed up toxin elimination and reduce post-workout inflammation.

Stretching and Mobility

Dedicating time to stretching and mobility exercises is crucial for maintaining flexibility and reducing injury risk. Specific mobility exercises improve joint range of motion and support the health of muscles and tendons.

Adequate Rest and Relaxation Techniques

Getting enough sleep is essential for recovery. Relaxation techniques, such as deep breathing, yoga, or meditation, reduce stress and help the body recover more efficiently. Relaxation supports overall recovery and prevents physical and mental burnout.

Tip: Dedicate at least one day a week to active recovery by incorporating stretching, mobility, and relaxation techniques to allow your body to fully recover.

How to Monitor Recovery: Signs of Overtraining and Prevention of Common Injuries

Monitoring recovery and watching for signs of overtraining are crucial to avoid burnout and injury. Here are some strategies to assess your recovery and prevent injuries:

Recognize Signs of Overtraining

Symptoms like persistent fatigue, lack of motivation, decreased performance, recurring pain, or sleep issues signal that the body needs more time to recover. Ignoring these signs can lead to serious injuries or mental exhaustion.

Adjust Training Load

Alternate intense training days with rest or low-intensity days. This allows the body to recover and prevents accumulated fatigue. You can also use a "progressive load" technique, gradually increasing training intensity.

Evaluate Your Sleep and Daily Energy Levels

Lack of sleep and low energy during the day indicate that the body is overloaded. Ensure you get 7–9 hours of sleep per night and listen to your body—if you feel exhausted, consider an active rest day.

Use Recovery Monitoring Tools

Apps and devices, such as heart rate monitors or activity trackers, can help you assess your resting heart rate and heart rate variability (HRV), indicators of nervous system recovery. A high resting heart rate may be a sign of overtraining.

Tip: Take time each week to assess your overall recovery and make adjustments to your training and supplementation routine. Listening to your body is the best way to prevent overtraining and injuries.

Nutrition and Supplementation for Cognitive Performance

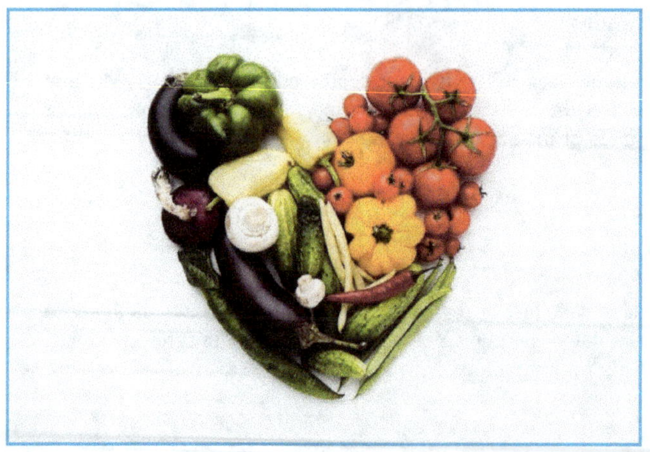

In a fast-paced world, maintaining optimal mental performance has become a priority for many. Mental clarity, concentration, and memory impact our work, studies, and daily activities, and are directly influenced by nutrition and lifestyle. This chapter focuses on how proper diet and supplementation can support cognitive function, improve memory, and strengthen mental resilience.

The Connection Between Nutrition and Cognitive Performance

Nutrition and cognitive performance are closely linked. The brain consumes about 20% of our daily energy, meaning that the food we eat plays a crucial role in its function. Macronutrients (carbohydrates, proteins, and fats) and micronutrients (vitamins and minerals) supply the brain with compounds necessary to maintain neural connections, reduce oxidative stress, and regulate neurotransmitters like dopamine and serotonin.

Complex Carbohydrates for Sustained Energy

The brain primarily relies on glucose for energy, so a low-carb diet can lead to decreased concentration and mental clarity. Eating complex carbohydrates, such as whole grains and legumes, provides a steady release of glucose, delivering continuous energy and avoiding sugar spikes and crashes.

Healthy Fats for Brain Health

Fats, especially omega-3 fatty acids, are essential structural components of brain cells. They improve neuron communication and help protect the brain from oxidative damage. Healthy fat sources include salmon, walnuts, olive oil, and avocado.

Proteins and Amino Acids for Neurotransmitters

Amino acids from proteins are precursors to neurotransmitters. For example, tryptophan is converted to serotonin, the mood-related neurotransmitter, and tyrosine is a precursor to dopamine, which is associated with motivation and focus. Complete proteins like those from animal sources, tofu, and quinoa are excellent options.

Tip: Keeping a balanced intake of macronutrients in each meal helps regulate energy levels and improve mental focus throughout the day.

Supplements for Concentration and Memory: Omega-3, Ginkgo Biloba, Ashwagandha, and Rhodiola

There are specific supplements that enhance concentration, memory, and mental clarity. Here are some of the most recommended:

Omega-3 (DHA and EPA)

Omega-3 fatty acids are essential for brain function. DHA, in particular, is a structural component of neuron membranes and enhances communication between brain cells. Studies show that omega-3s can improve memory and cognitive processing speed, especially in older adults.

Recommended Dose: 250–500 mg of combined DHA and EPA daily.

Ginkgo Biloba

Ginkgo biloba is a natural supplement known for improving blood circulation in the brain. By increasing blood flow, it enhances oxygen and nutrient supply, helping to improve memory and concentration.

Recommended Dose: 120–240 mg daily, ideally split into two doses.

Ashwagandha

Ashwagandha is an adaptogen that reduces stress and enhances mental resilience. It lowers cortisol, a stress hormone that affects memory and concentration. Ashwagandha is ideal for those seeking mental and emotional support during demanding periods.

Recommended Dose: 300–600 mg of standardized ashwagandha root extract daily.

Rhodiola Rosea

Another popular adaptogen, Rhodiola rosea, is known for improving mood and stress resistance. Studies have shown that it helps reduce mental fatigue and enhances focus for individuals facing prolonged stress.

Recommended Dose: 200–400 mg daily, ideally before activities requiring high concentration.

Tip: Combining adaptogens like ashwagandha and Rhodiola with omega-3s creates a synergy that supports both brain function and stress resilience.

Essential Micronutrients for the Brain: Importance of B Vitamins, Magnesium, and Zinc

Micronutrients are essential for the brain, as they support energy production and neurotransmitter function. Here are some of the most important ones:

B Vitamins (Especially B6, B9, and B12)

B vitamins are crucial for energy production in brain cells and aid in neurotransmitter synthesis. Vitamin B12, in particular, protects against cognitive decline and improves memory. A deficiency in these vitamins can negatively impact concentration and mood.

Recommended Dose: You can take B-complex supplements to cover daily recommended intake or adjust the dosage according to specific deficiencies.

Magnesium

Magnesium regulates nerve function and helps reduce stress and anxiety, promoting relaxation without affecting mental clarity. It's especially useful for those who need stress relief without losing focus.

Recommended Dose: 300–400 mg daily, preferably in the evening.

Zinc

Zinc is an essential mineral for memory and learning. Deficiency can impair cognitive capacity and affect mood. It helps protect the brain from oxidative damage and supports neurotransmitter function.

Recommended Dose: 10–20 mg daily, ideally taken with a main meal.

Tip: Make sure to obtain these micronutrients from a varied diet, and if needed, supplement them according to your specific needs with professional guidance.

Tips to Optimize Cognitive Performance

Beyond nutrition and supplementation, certain habits and practices can help you optimize cognitive performance and maintain an active, alert mind.

Establish a Reading Habit

Reading regularly improves concentration and stimulates different areas of the brain. Spend at least 20–30 minutes a day reading books, articles, or topics that interest you.

Practice Meditation

Meditation strengthens focus, reduces stress, and improves mental clarity. By practicing meditation, the brain learns to ignore distractions, which improves concentration in other areas of life.

Get Adequate Rest

Sleep is crucial for the brain as it allows memory consolidation and cognitive recovery. During sleep, the brain processes information from the day and strengthens neural connections. Sleeping 7–9 hours daily is ideal for optimal mental performance.

Engage in Regular Physical Exercise

Physical activity improves blood circulation, delivering more oxygen to the brain and stimulating the growth of new brain cells. Aerobic exercise and strength training are excellent for mental health and cognition.

Tip: Combine these habits to maintain a routine that nurtures your mind and reduces stress. Consistency in these practices can enhance the effects of supplementation and nutrition.

Balanced Nutrition for Brain Health: Sample Day of Eating for Mental Well-being

A balanced, nutrient-rich diet is essential for cognitive performance. Here is an example of a day's meal plan that provides nutrients to support brain function.

Breakfast

Oatmeal with walnuts, chia seeds, and berries: Oats provide complex carbs, walnuts and chia seeds are rich in omega-3s, and berries contain antioxidants that protect brain cells.

Coffee or green tea. Both contain caffeine, which improves attention, and antioxidants that protect the brain.

Lunch

Spinach, quinoa, avocado, and salmon salad: Spinach is rich in B vitamins, salmon provides omega-3s, and quinoa is a source of slow-release carbs to maintain energy levels.

Olive oil and lemon dressing: Olive oil offers healthy fats that benefit brain function.

Mid-afternoon Snack

Natural yogurt with blueberries and almonds: Yogurt is a source of probiotics that support the gut-brain axis. Blueberries and almonds provide antioxidants and healthy fats.

Dinner

Baked chicken with sweet potatoes and steamed broccoli: Chicken provides protein for neurotransmitters, while sweet potatoes and broccoli supply complex carbs and vitamin C, helping to reduce oxidative stress.

Before Bed

Tip: Incorporating nutrient-dense, balanced foods throughout the day is key to sustaining continuous cognitive performance and enhancing mental well-being.

Meal Planning and Preparation to Support Supplementation

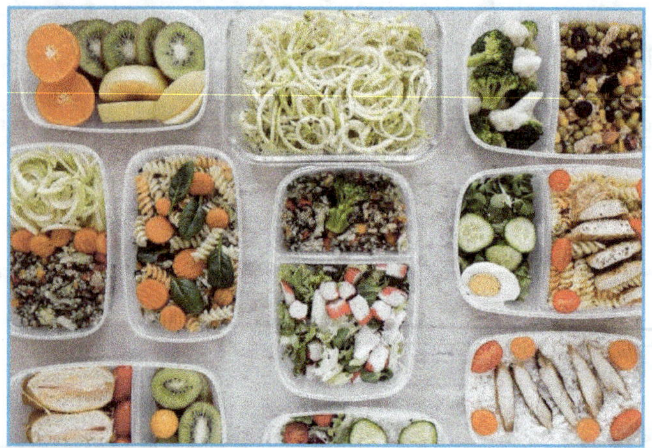

Meal planning not only makes it easier to follow a balanced diet but can also enhance the effects of the supplements you take. By strategically combining certain foods with your supplements, you help your body absorb and utilize nutrients more effectively. This chapter will guide you in creating a meal plan that optimizes supplementation, with practical recipe ideas and meal-prep tips that align with your physical and mental performance goals.

How to Combine Supplements with Foods to Optimize Absorption

Some supplements are better absorbed when combined with specific foods. Taking advantage of these principles can make a significant difference in the effectiveness of your supplementation. Here's how to improve the absorption of some common supplements:

Vitamin D and Coenzyme Q10 with Healthy Fats

Both vitamin D and coenzyme Q10 are fat-soluble, meaning their absorption improves in the presence of fats. Consuming these supplements alongside a meal with avocado, olive oil, nuts, or salmon can increase their effectiveness.

Example: Take vitamin D at breakfast with avocado toast or a smoothie containing coconut oil.

Iron with Vitamin C

Iron absorbs better when paired with vitamin C. If you're taking an iron supplement, pair it with vitamin C-rich fruits like strawberries, oranges, or kiwi.

Example: Take your iron supplement with a smoothie made from berries or a glass of orange juice.

Calcium and Magnesium at Different Times of Day

Calcium and magnesium are essential for bone and muscle health but compete for absorption in the intestines. For maximum effectiveness, consume calcium during the day (with a meal) and take magnesium at night, ideally before bedtime to promote relaxation.

Omega-3 with Meals

Omega-3 fatty acids are better absorbed when taken with foods, especially those containing healthy fats. Taking your omega-3 supplement with a meal high in healthy fats, like a salad with olive oil or a fish dish, improves its bioavailability.

Example: Take your omega-3 supplement with lunch or dinner, paired with a healthy fat source.

Tip: Plan the timing and food pairings of your supplements for optimal effectiveness. Always consult a healthcare professional if you have questions about supplement combinations.

Creating a Weekly Meal Plan

A weekly plan ensures you consume all the nutrients you need and helps you stay on track with your supplementation plan. Here's a step-by-step guide for creating a balanced meal plan:

Define Your Nutritional Goals

Start by clarifying your goal: Are you looking to enhance physical performance, build muscle, reduce body fat, or improve general health? This will determine your macronutrient distribution and choice of supplements.

Select Sources of Protein, Carbohydrates, and Fats

Include a high-quality protein source in each meal (chicken, fish, eggs, legumes), complex carbohydrates for sustained energy (brown rice, sweet potatoes, quinoa), and healthy fats (avocado, nuts, olive oil).

Incorporate Foods Rich in Vitamins and Minerals

Ensure a variety of fruits and vegetables for a wide range of vitamins and minerals. Foods like spinach, carrots, blueberries, and peppers are excellent options for balanced nutrition that enhances your supplementation.

Sample Weekly Plan

Monday

Breakfast: Protein smoothie with spinach, banana, and almond milk (with vitamin D supplement).

Lunch: Salmon quinoa salad with avocado and spinach (with omega-3).

Dinner: Baked chicken breast with sweet potatoes and broccoli.

Tuesday

Breakfast: Oatmeal with berries, chia seeds, and nuts.

Lunch: Roast turkey with brown rice and roasted vegetables.

Dinner: Grilled fish fillet with cauliflower mash and green salad.

Prepara snacks y comidas adicionales

Include healthy snacks like fresh fruits, Greek yogurt with nuts, or carrot sticks with hummus. This ensures you have nutritious options between meals and helps maintain a steady nutrient supply.

Tip: Take time on Sundays to plan your meals and make a shopping list. This simplifies your week and ensures every meal aligns with your nutritional and supplementation goals.

Practical Recipes for Health and Performance

Here are some easy, practical recipes that not only add flavor but also enhance physical and mental performance:

Breakfast: Avocado Toast with Eggs and Spinach

Ingredients: 1 avocado, 2 eggs, 1 cup fresh spinach, 2 slices whole-grain bread.

Instructions: Toast the bread and spread avocado slices on each slice. Cook eggs to preference and place them on top of the avocado. Sauté spinach and add it to the plate. Ideal with vitamin D and omega-3 supplements.

Lunch: Quinoa Salad with Salmon, Walnuts, and Asparagus

Ingredients: 1 cup cooked quinoa, 1 grilled salmon fillet, 1/4 cup walnuts, steamed asparagus, fresh spinach, olive oil, and lemon.

Instructions: Place quinoa in a bowl, add shredded salmon, walnuts, and asparagus. Dress with olive oil and lemon. Perfect for boosting coenzyme Q10 and omega-3 absorption.

Dinner: Lettuce Tacos with Lemon Chicken and Avocado

Ingredients: 1 chicken breast cut into strips, romaine lettuce leaves, 1 avocado, lemon juice, salt, and pepper.

Instructions: Cook chicken strips with lemon juice, salt, and pepper. Fill lettuce leaves with chicken and top with avocado slices. This light dinner pairs well with magnesium for better recovery and rest.

Tip: These recipes are nutrient-dense, easy to prepare, and effectively complement any supplementation regimen.

Meal Prep Tips

Meal prep is a powerful tool for maintaining a balanced diet, saving time, and supporting supplementation. Here are some techniques for organizing your weekly meals:

Plan and Make a Shopping List

Define your recipes for the week and create a detailed list of ingredients. This will save you time at the grocery store and help you stay focused on your nutrition goals.

Cook in Large Batches

Prepare proteins, carbohydrates, and vegetables in large quantities. For example, cook several servings of rice, chicken breasts, and steamed vegetables. Store each ingredient in separate containers for easy combination throughout the week.

Portion Out Your Meals

Use individual containers to divide meals into portions, which makes it easier to control portion sizes and ensures each meal is balanced and ready to eat.

Freeze as Needed

If you're preparing meals for the entire week, freeze the ones you won't eat in the first few days to maintain freshness. Thaw them the night before to enjoy them at their best.

Tip: Dedicate a couple of hours to meal prep on Sundays. This time investment ensures your meals are ready, reducing the temptation to eat out and making sure each meal supports your supplementation plan.

Healthy Snack Options to Boost Energy and Recovery

Snacks are a great way to maintain energy levels and support recovery between main meals. Here are some healthy options that complement your supplementation and are easy to prepare:

Greek Yogurt with Berries and Chia Seeds

High in protein and antioxidants, this snack supports muscle recovery and digestive health.

Turkey Strips with Hummus and Carrot Sticks

Rich in protein and fiber, this snack is excellent for curbing hunger and maintaining energy throughout the day.

Protein Smoothie with Spinach, Banana, and Almond Butter

This smoothie is ideal as a pre- or post-workout snack, combining protein with quick-absorbing carbs to support muscle recovery.

Nuts and Dried Fruit

Nuts provide healthy fats, while dried fruit offers quick-absorbing carbs. This snack is portable and maintains energy without causing a sugar spike.

Tip: Keep some of these snacks prepared during the week to avoid hunger spikes and sustain your energy levels throughout the day.

Supplementation for Different Types of Training

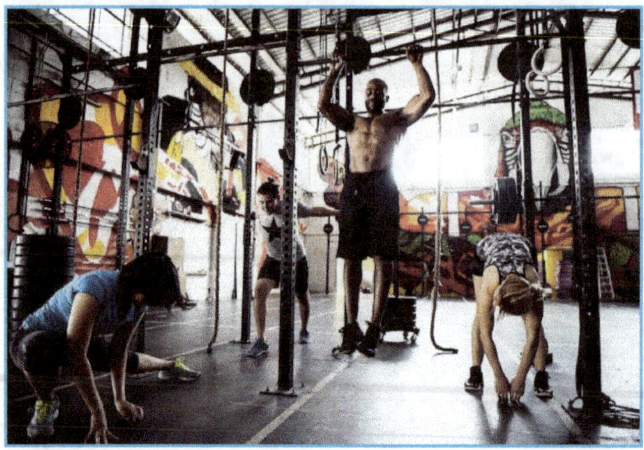

Each type of training places unique demands on the body, so choosing the right supplements should align with the specific needs of the activity. Whether you're training for strength, endurance, or flexibility, there are supplements that can enhance your performance and recovery. This chapter will guide you through the most suitable supplements for each type of training to help you optimize results based on your goals.

Strength and Muscle Endurance Training

Strength and muscle endurance training includes activities like weightlifting, resistance band workouts, and muscle hypertrophy work. The goal is to increase strength, power, and muscle size, so supplements that support protein synthesis, muscle recovery, and energy production are especially beneficial.

Creatine

Creatine is one of the most researched and effective supplements for boosting strength and performance in high-intensity, short-duration exercises. It helps increase ATP production, the energy source muscles use for lifting, and supports muscle mass gain.

Recommended Dose: Loading phase of 20g per day for 5-7 days, followed by a maintenance dose of 3-5g daily.

Protein (Whey, Casein, Plant Protein)

Protein is essential for muscle synthesis and post-workout recovery. Sufficient protein intake reduces muscle breakdown and promotes lean muscle gain. Whey protein is ideal for post-workout as it absorbs quickly, while casein is an excellent option before bed due to its slow digestion rate.

Recommended Dose: 20-30g of protein powder after training or 1.6-2.2g/kg of body weight distributed throughout the day.

BCAA (Branched-Chain Amino Acids)

BCAAs (leucine, isoleucine, and valine) help reduce muscle fatigue and improve recovery. They are especially useful if you train on an empty stomach or have long workout sessions, as they provide essential amino acids directly to muscles.

Recommended Dose: 5-10g before or after training, depending on needs and session duration.

Tip: Combine creatine and BCAAs to maximize strength and recovery, and ensure you consume quality protein within a few hours after training.

Endurance Training (Cardio, Long Distance)

Endurance training includes long-duration cardiovascular activities like running, cycling, and swimming. This type of training requires a constant energy source and electrolytes to maintain hydration and prevent fatigue. Here are key supplements for endurance:

Electrolytes

Electrolytes (sodium, potassium, magnesium, and calcium) help maintain fluid balance, prevent muscle cramps, and are essential for those training for long periods and sweating heavily.

Recommended Dose: 500-1000mg of sodium and 200-400mg of potassium per hour of intense activity, adjusted for sweat levels.

Fast-Absorbing Carbohydrates

Fast-absorbing carbs, like maltodextrin or dextrose, are ideal for maintaining blood glucose levels and providing immediate energy during endurance training. They help prevent fatigue and sustain performance.

Recommended Dose: 30-60g of carbs per hour during workouts longer than 90 minutes.

Beta-Alanine

Beta-alanine helps delay lactic acid buildup in muscles, allowing prolonged effort. This supplement is particularly useful for high-intensity endurance training, like long-distance cycling and running.

Recommended Dose: 3-6g daily, divided into doses of 1-2g to prevent tingling sensation.

Tip: During endurance training, alternate between electrolytes and quick-absorbing carbs to maintain energy and hydration, helping prevent exhaustion and sustain performance throughout the session.

HIIT and CrossFit Training

High-intensity interval training (HIIT) and CrossFit combine strength and endurance exercises in short but intense sessions. These modalities require supplements that help maximize energy and recovery, as wear and tear is high in each session.

Caffeine

Caffeine is a stimulant that increases alertness, reduces perceived effort, and boosts performance in high-intensity exercises. Taking it before a HIIT or CrossFit workout can improve power and endurance during intervals.

Recommended Dose: 3-6mg of caffeine per kg of body weight, around 30-60 minutes before training.

Fast-Absorbing Protein and Carbs

Since HIIT and CrossFit demand quick recovery, consuming a source of protein and carbohydrates post-workout helps replenish glycogen stores and initiate muscle repair.

Recommended Dose: 20-30g of protein with 30-50g of fast-absorbing carbs post-workout.

Electrolytes

Like in endurance training, HIIT and CrossFit lead to significant fluid and electrolyte loss due to intense sweating. Maintaining electrolyte balance is crucial to prevent cramps and stay hydrated.

Recommended Dose: 500-1000mg of sodium along with potassium and magnesium, depending on training duration and intensity.

Tip: Take a pre-workout with caffeine and ensure you replenish protein and carbs after training to maximize energy and enhance muscle recovery.

Yoga, Pilates, and Flexibility Sports

Yoga, Pilates, and other flexibility-focused sports emphasize mobility, core strength, and joint health. Although not high-intensity, these exercises benefit from supplements that promote joint health, relaxation, and recovery from physical stress.

Collagen

Collagen is a protein that helps maintain joint elasticity and connective tissue strength. Consuming collagen improves joint health and strengthens tendons, which is essential in activities requiring a high range of motion.

Recommended Dose: 10-15g of hydrolyzed collagen daily, ideally with a vitamin C source for better absorption.

Magnesium

Magnesium is essential for muscle relaxation and nerve function. Taking magnesium after training helps reduce muscle tension, making it ideal for those practicing flexibility sports.

Recommended Dose: 300-400mg daily, ideally at night to promote relaxation and sleep.

Ashwagandha

Ashwagandha is an adaptogen that helps reduce stress and improves mental resilience. This supplement is especially beneficial for those seeking a yoga or Pilates practice oriented toward mental wellness, as it lowers cortisol and supports a calm state.

Recommended Dose: 300-600mg of standardized ashwagandha root extract daily.

Tip: Incorporate collagen and magnesium to optimize recovery and reduce joint and muscle stiffness, enhancing the quality of your flexibility sessions.

Supplementation Examples by Training Type: Recommended Dosages and Timing

Here are specific examples of how and when to take certain supplements based on the type of training:

Strength Training

Before: 5g of creatine and 5g of BCAAs.

After: 20-30g of whey protein and 3-5g of creatine (if not taken before).

Endurance Training

During: 500-1000mg of electrolytes and 30-60g of carbs per hour (if a long session).

After: 20-30g of protein and 1-2g of beta-alanine.

HIIT/CrossFit Training

Before: 3-6mg of caffeine per kg of body weight and 5g of BCAAs.

After: 20-30g of whey protein and 30-50g of fast-absorbing carbs.

Yoga/Pilates

Before: 5-10g of hydrolyzed collagen and a vitamin C source.

After: 300-400mg of magnesium in the evening for better recovery and rest.

Tip: Adjust the dose and timing of each supplement according to your specific needs and goals. The key is to adapt to the demands of your training and ensure the body has the necessary support to perform at its best and recover efficiently.

Myths and Realities about Supplementation

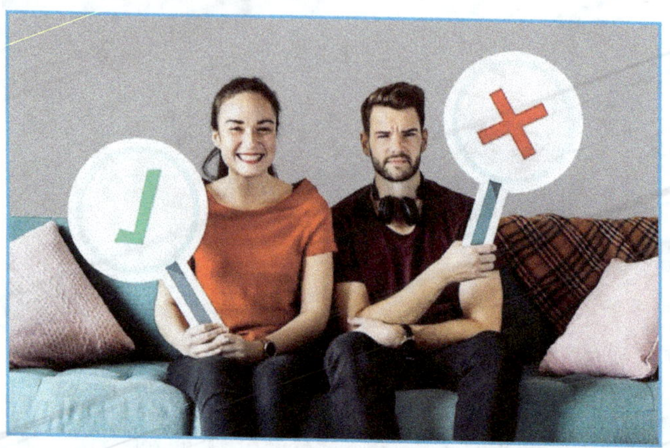

Supplementation is a field full of promises, and in many cases, exaggerations. As the supplement industry has grown, so have the myths and misconceptions, often fueled by marketing strategies that exploit people's needs and desires. To make informed decisions and reap real benefits from supplements, it's essential to distinguish between what's scientifically supported and what's just unsubstantiated advertising. This chapter addresses some of the most common myths, what science says, and how to avoid misleading marketing to make smart purchasing choices.

Popular Supplements: Myth or Reality?

Here, we break down some of the most popular supplements and evaluate whether their claimed benefits are backed by science or simply marketing hype.

Multivitamins

Myth: "Multivitamins are essential to meet all your nutritional needs."

Reality: For many people with a balanced diet, multivitamins are not strictly necessary, as most nutritional requirements can be met through a varied diet. However, they can be helpful for people with dietary restrictions, like vegans or those with nutrient absorption issues.

Scientific Evidence: Some studies suggest that multivitamins don't offer significant benefits in preventing chronic diseases for those with a healthy diet. However, they can help prevent specific deficiencies in high-risk groups, such as older adults and people with restrictive diets.

BCAA (Branched-Chain Amino Acids)

Myth: "BCAAs are essential for muscle growth and post-exercise recovery."

Reality: If you consume enough protein in your diet (from whole foods or supplements), additional BCAAs don't typically offer significant benefits for muscle growth. BCAAs are three of the nine essential amino acids present in complete proteins, so their effect is redundant if the diet is already high in protein.

Scientific Evidence: Studies indicate that complete protein supplements (like whey or casein) are more effective for recovery and muscle growth, as they provide all essential amino acids, not just BCAAs.

Collagen

Myth: "Collagen improves skin, joint health, and slows aging."

Reality: Collagen is a protein naturally found in the body and breaks down into amino acids during digestion. Although the body can use these amino acids to create collagen, there's no guarantee they'll specifically benefit the skin or joints.

Scientific Evidence: Preliminary evidence suggests that collagen may improve skin elasticity and joint health in some cases, but its effectiveness varies by individual and product quality. For those interested in joint health, other well-supported supplements like glucosamine and MSM are also available.

Fat Burners

Myth: "Fat burners speed up metabolism and help you lose weight quickly."

Reality: "Fat burners" usually contain caffeine and other stimulants that can temporarily increase energy expenditure, but their effect on weight loss is minimal. Sustainable weight loss still primarily depends on a proper diet and regular exercise.

Scientific Evidence: Most fat burner ingredients lack sufficient evidence to support their claims. Effects are generally mild and temporary, and these products may pose risks, such as increased blood pressure and anxiety.

Vitamin C for the Immune System

Myth: "Vitamin C prevents colds and other illnesses by strengthening the immune system."

Reality: While vitamin C is important for immune health, high doses of vitamin C have not been shown to prevent colds for most people. However, it may reduce the duration and severity of symptoms for those with a deficiency or low regular intake of vitamin C.

Scientific Evidence: Studies suggest that vitamin C supplementation only moderately reduces the duration of the common cold in certain people, especially athletes or those under intense stress.

What Science Supports vs. Popular Beliefs

Some supplements have well-documented effects supported by solid scientific evidence, while others are marketed with exaggerated claims without conclusive proof. Let's look at what science backs:

Protein Powder

Protein powder is scientifically supported to aid in muscle recovery and lean mass gain, especially for active people who don't meet their daily protein needs through diet alone. Whey protein, in particular, is a high-quality, fast-absorbing source ideal for post-workout consumption.

Creatine

Creatine is one of the most studied supplements and has proven effective for improving strength, power, and performance in high-intensity sports. It also helps increase muscle mass and aids in recovery. Its safety and efficacy have been confirmed across various studies, and since it isn't a stimulant, it can be used over the long term without significant side effects for most people.

Omega-3 (EPA and DHA)

Omega-3 fatty acids have scientific support for their benefits on cardiovascular health, brain function, and anti-inflammatory effects. Omega-3s are essential because the body cannot produce them, and studies show that a diet high in omega-3s reduces the risk of heart disease and improves cognitive function.

Vitamin D

Vitamin D is essential for bone health, immune function, and mood regulation. Deficiency in vitamin D is common due to lack of sunlight exposure, and supplementation has been shown to improve overall health, especially for those with deficiencies.

Magnesium

Magnesium is essential for muscle and nerve function, sleep regulation, and energy production. Its deficiency can cause muscle cramps, fatigue, and sleep issues, and supplementation can help alleviate these symptoms, especially in active individuals.

How to Avoid Falling for Misleading Marketing and Buy Smartly

The supplement industry generates billions of dollars annually, and companies often make bold claims to attract buyers. Learning to identify misleading marketing will help you avoid spending money on unnecessary or ineffective products. Here are some strategies for informed supplement shopping:

Research Ingredients and Their Effects

Don't be swayed by claims like "natural," "revolutionary," or "clinically proven." Research the main ingredients and look for studies that support their benefits. Scientific information is available in peer-reviewed journals and reputable health websites.

Be Wary of Exaggerated Claims

Supplements promising quick results, like "weight loss in 7 days" or "muscle gain in a week," tend to exaggerate their effects or even use harmful ingredients. Weight loss and muscle growth are gradual processes that don't happen overnight.

Choose Quality-Certified Products

Look for supplements with quality certifications from third-party organizations, such as NSF International, USP, or GMP (Good Manufacturing Practices). These certifications indicate that the product has been tested for purity, potency, and quality and is safe for consumption.

Avoid "Miracle" Supplements

Some products are marketed as a "miracle cure" for a wide range of issues. Be skeptical of any supplement claiming to be a solution for multiple health problems, as it's unlikely that a single product can effectively address various conditions.

Read Reviews from Trusted Sources

While online reviews can be helpful, it's important to read opinions from trusted sources, such as health and nutrition websites or experts in the field. Reviews on sales sites can be manipulated, so it's best to research across different platforms.

Consult a Professional Before Starting a New Supplement

A nutritionist or healthcare professional can help you select supplements you actually need and that align with your goals and lifestyle. They can also recommend a proper dosage and monitor your progress, preventing any potential adverse effects or interactions with other supplements or medications.

Final Considerations and Planning Your Supplementation

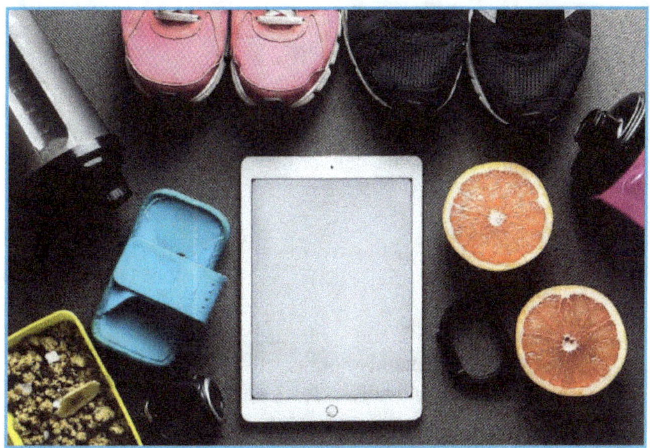

Supplementation can be a powerful ally on your journey toward optimal health, but its success greatly depends on careful planning, ongoing evaluation, and commitment to a healthy lifestyle. This chapter brings together best practices to help you start supplementing safely, adapt your plan to meet changing needs, and access reliable sources of information to stay well-informed.

How to Track Your Results

A key aspect of knowing if your supplementation plan is working is tracking your results. Changes may be subtle and not always noticeable initially, so recording your progress can help you see improvements and make adjustments as needed. Here are some effective ways to track:

Set Measurable Goals

Define specific goals from the start. For example, if you're taking a protein supplement to gain muscle mass, set a target in terms of strength, muscle size, or body weight. If you're taking melatonin to improve sleep, measure sleep quality and duration over weeks or months.

Record Symptoms and Well-being

Keep a symptom journal or wellness log where you can note changes in energy levels, mood, digestion, or sleep quality. This is especially useful for supplements that impact general well-being, such as magnesium, ashwagandha, or omega-3.

Measure Physical Progress

For supplements related to physical performance, use specific metrics like weight lifted, reps, recovery time, or endurance in cardio activities. This allows you to see if performance supplements, like creatine or BCAAs, are delivering results.

Do Lab Tests

Some supplements, such as vitamin D, vitamin B12, and iron, can be monitored through blood tests. Conducting tests before and after several months of supplementation can help confirm if your levels are in the ideal range and adjust doses as needed.

Be Patient and Consistent

Remember that supplement results aren't instant. Many require several weeks or months to show visible benefits. Consistency is key: follow a regular regimen and give your body time to adapt.

Recommendations for Starting Supplementation Safely

Safety is crucial when beginning a supplementation plan. Start with the right approach to avoid issues such as overdosing or unwanted interactions.

Consult a Professional

Before starting any supplements, consult a nutritionist or doctor, especially if you have pre-existing health conditions or take medications. A professional can guide you on the appropriate doses and the types of supplements you actually need.

Start with Low Doses and Adjust Gradually

If it's your first time taking a supplement, begin with the lowest recommended dose and observe how your body responds. This is especially important with stimulating supplements, like caffeine, to avoid side effects like nervousness or anxiety.

Avoid Starting Too Many Supplements at Once

Introducing many supplements simultaneously can make it hard to track individual effects and increases the risk of interactions. Start one supplement at a time, allowing two to four weeks before adding another to observe its effects.

Read Labels and Ensure Product Purity

Not all supplements are equal in quality and purity. Choose products from reputable brands with quality certifications like NSF, USP, or GMP, which ensure that the product meets safety standards and contains the ingredients listed on the label.

Stay Hydrated and Maintain a Balanced Diet

Supplements are an aid, but food remains the foundation. Follow a balanced diet and drink plenty of water to support the absorption and metabolism of supplements.

How to Adapt Your Supplementation Over Time

As your goals, needs, and health status change, your supplementation plan may also need adjustments. Adapting supplementation allows you to maximize its benefits throughout your life.

Review Your Supplement Plan Every 3 to 6 Months

Effective supplementation is dynamic. Assess every so often to see if you're meeting your goals and if adjustments are needed. This is especially useful if your goals change, such as shifting from muscle gain to general health improvement.

Adjust According to Lifestyle and Season

Some supplements may be more necessary at certain times of the year. For example, in winter, vitamin D is often needed more due to lower sun exposure. If you increase training intensity, you might need more protein or electrolytes for recovery support.

Listen to Your Body

If you notice side effects like slow digestion, insomnia, or anxiety, consider adjusting the dose or eliminating the problematic supplement. Not all supplements work the same for everyone; personalize your supplementation based on what works best for you.

Monitor Results in Light of Health Changes and Aging

As you age, your nutritional needs change. Older adults may need more vitamin D, calcium, and magnesium for bone support, while growing adolescents may need additional iron and protein. Adjusting supplementation to each life stage is key to maintaining health.

Reliable Sources of Information and Current Studies

With so much information available online, it's essential to rely on credible and evidence-based sources to make informed supplementation decisions. Here are some sources and tips for evaluating information quality:

Peer-Reviewed Scientific Publications

Access scientific databases like PubMed or Google Scholar for studies reviewed by experts in the field. These publications provide direct evidence on the effectiveness and safety of each supplement.

Trusted Health Institutions

Organizations like the Mayo Clinic, National Institutes of Health (NIH), World Health Organization (WHO), and National Health Service (NHS) are reliable sources that provide expert-backed, updated information.

Certified Nutrition and Medical Professionals

Nutritionists and doctors experienced in supplementation can offer personalized, evidence-based recommendations. Many also share information on blogs and social media, but ensure they are accredited and use a scientific approach.

Specialized Health and Nutrition Journals

Publications like The American Journal of Clinical Nutrition and The Journal of Nutrition publish reliable studies and reviews on supplementation. These journals specialize in health and nutrition topics and are often excellent sources of updated information.

Consult Systematic Reviews and Meta-Analyses

Systematic reviews and meta-analyses examine the results of multiple studies on a specific topic, providing a comprehensive overview of available evidence. These reviews are useful for an objective view of a supplement's effectiveness.

Frequently Asked Questions

To conclude, here are answers to some common questions about supplementation:

Is it necessary to take supplements if I have a balanced diet?

Not necessarily. A complete, balanced diet can cover most nutritional needs, but some supplements can be beneficial for certain people (e.g., vitamin B12 for vegans or vitamin D for those in cold climates).

Can I take multiple supplements at once?

Yes, you can combine supplements, but it's important to introduce one at a time and understand each one's possible effects. Additionally, some supplements may interfere with each other's absorption, so it's helpful to space them out or consult a professional.

How long should I take a supplement to see results?

This varies by supplement and goal. Some, like caffeine, produce immediate effects, while others, like vitamin D or CoQ10, require several weeks or even months of consistent use to show significant benefits.

Is it safe to take supplements long-term?

Generally, yes, as long as recommended doses are followed and unnecessary supplements are avoided. However, it's important to evaluate the need for each supplement and adjust doses according to professional recommendations.

What are the best supplements to start with?

This depends on individual needs, but the most common include a quality multivitamin, vitamin D for low sun exposure, omega-3 for cardiovascular health, and protein for growth and muscle recovery in active individuals.

Additional Resources and Bibliography

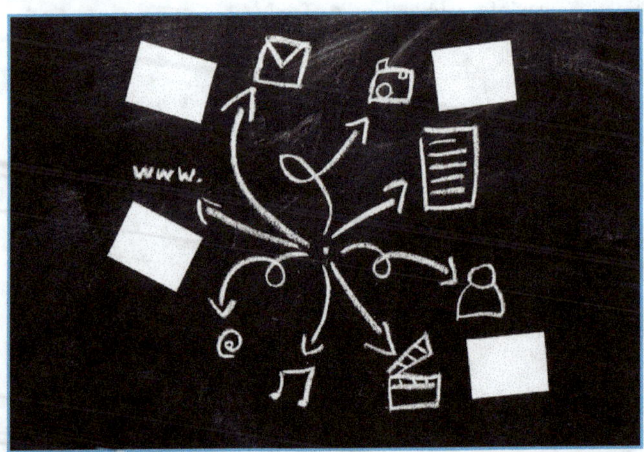

The world of supplementation, nutrition, and fitness is constantly evolving, and staying informed with reliable sources is essential for achieving results safely and effectively. This chapter provides a list of scientific references, websites, apps, and recommended readings so you can deepen your understanding of the topic and optimize the tracking of your goals.

Scientific References and Recommended Readings

Scientific research is the foundation for understanding the efficacy and safety of supplements. Here is a list of journals and studies that frequently address topics related to supplementation, nutrition, and physical performance.

Peer-Reviewed Scientific Publications

These journals and scientific databases publish studies on nutrition, supplementation, and sports medicine, providing reliable and up-to-date scientific evidence on the effectiveness of various supplements:

The American Journal of Clinical Nutrition: Publishes original research and reviews on nutrition topics, including the impact of supplements on health.

The Journal of the International Society of Sports Nutrition (JISSN): Focuses on research related to sports nutrition, including the use of supplements for performance.

PubMed: A free database of medical and scientific research. You can search for specific studies on supplements and nutrition.

The New England Journal of Medicine (NEJM): One of the most prestigious medical journals, often publishing studies and reviews on health and nutrition topics.

Key Scientific Articles on Supplementation

Some studies have made significant contributions to our understanding of certain supplements. Here are some of the most influential ones:

Creatine Supplementation and Exercise Performance: A study that establishes the effectiveness of creatine in increasing strength and power.

Vitamin D Supplementation and Muscle Function: A review on the effects of vitamin D on bone and muscle health.

The Effects of Fish Oil on Heart Health: A meta-analysis on the benefits of omega-3 for cardiovascular health.

Systematic Reviews and Meta-Analyses

Systematic reviews and meta-analyses combine results from multiple studies to offer a comprehensive and well-supported view on a specific topic. These studies are particularly useful for controversial topics or those with mixed evidence. You can find relevant reviews on:

- Effects of caffeine on sports performance
- Benefits and risks of antioxidants
- Impact of magnesium on sleep and stress management

Using digital tools can help you accurately track your progress and optimize your fitness, health, and supplementation goals. Below are reliable websites and apps for monitoring and planning.

Trusted Websites

Examine.com: Specializes in researching the effectiveness and safety of supplements. Publishes study summaries on hundreds of supplements, providing an unbiased, evidence-based analysis.

MyFitnessPal: A food and macros tracking platform. You can record your nutrient intake and monitor calorie, protein, fat, and carbohydrate needs, which is essential for optimizing supplementation.

National Institutes of Health (NIH) - Office of Dietary Supplements: Provides unbiased information on various supplements, their effects, and recommended dosages.

Labdoor: Tests the purity and quality of commercial supplements, ranking them based on effectiveness and safety. It's helpful for those who want to ensure their supplements are safe and contain what they claim.

Apps for Monitoring and Tracking

Cronometer: An advanced food tracking app that provides a detailed breakdown of micronutrients, as well as macronutrients. Ideal for people looking to ensure adequate vitamin and mineral intake alongside their supplements.

Fitbod: This training app customizes your routines based on progress and fitness level. It allows you to plan supplementation according to training and rest days.

Sleep Cycle: Monitoring sleep quality is essential, especially if you're taking supplements to improve rest (like melatonin or magnesium). This app analyzes your sleep patterns and helps you optimize your nighttime routine.

Athlytic (for Apple Watch users): Provides data on recovery, stress, and physical performance, helping you know when you might need additional support from certain supplements, like protein or adaptogens.

Online Calculators

Caloric and Macronutrient Requirement Calculators, such as Precision Nutrition or IIFYM's Macro Calculator, help you set daily nutrition goals and complement your diet with the right supplements.

Water and Electrolyte Needs Calculators: Useful for those who train at high intensity and need to optimize hydration, especially when taking supplements like creatine.

Books and Articles for In-Depth Understanding

For those who want a deeper understanding of supplementation, nutrition, and fitness, there are books and articles that offer extensive, evidence-based information in an accessible way. Below are some recommendations:

Books on Supplementation and Sports Nutrition

Supplements: The Ultimate Supplement Guide for Men by Mike Matthews: Offers a clear, practical guide on the most useful supplements for men seeking to improve their health and physical performance.

Nutritional Supplements in Sports and Exercise by Ira Wolinsky and Judy Driskell: This book addresses the scientific evidence behind sports supplements and their practical application for performance.

The Complete Guide to Sports Nutrition by Anita Bean: A comprehensive guide on sports nutrition covering the basic principles of supplementation and its application in the context of performance and health.

The Endurance Diet by Matt Fitzgerald: Aimed at endurance athletes, this book explains how to optimize nutrition for recovery and performance through appropriate supplementation.

Digital Articles and Resources

How to Make Sense of Supplement Research: An article by Examine.com that explains how to read scientific studies on supplements and evaluate their validity.

The Athlete's Guide to Sports Supplements from the American College of Sports Medicine: A guide on the use of supplements in high-performance sports. Covers topics like hydration, electrolyte balance, and recovery support supplements.

ConsumerLab: A paid platform that offers unbiased reviews and lab analyses of various supplements on the market, including guides on effectiveness, purity, and recommended dosages.

Educational Podcasts and Blogs

The Drive by Peter Attia: This podcast addresses topics on longevity, metabolic health, and supplementation from a scientific perspective. Many episodes focus on the impact of certain nutrients and supplements on long-term health.

FoundMyFitness by Rhonda Patrick: A podcast and blog that explore health and nutrition topics based on scientific research, including specific episodes on vitamin D, omega-3, and other key supplements.

Sigma Nutrition Radio: Hosted by Danny Lennon, this podcast focuses on evidence-based nutrition. Many episodes analyze the use of supplements and their impact on sports performance and general health.

How to Evaluate Sources of Information on Supplementation

It's essential to learn to identify and evaluate reliable sources of information on supplementation to avoid falling into marketing hype or inaccurate information. Here are some guidelines to ensure the information you're consuming is high-quality:

Look for Credible Authors
Make sure the author or source of the information has credentials and training in nutrition, medicine, or exercise science. Check if the content has been reviewed by experts or is based on studies published in scientific journals.

Consult Peer-Reviewed Studies
Peer-reviewed research is the foundation of reliable science. Look for information in databases like PubMed, Google Scholar, or ResearchGate, where you can read summaries of studies and full articles.

Check the References of Claims
Reliable sources usually back up their claims with references to scientific studies. Be wary of articles that lack references or only cite other blogs or websites without scientific support.

Avoid Sources with Conflicts of Interest
Many supplement brands publish "information" that's actually marketing disguised as science. Look for independent sources and consider conflicts of interest before taking the information seriously.

Stay Updated
Supplementation science is constantly evolving. Keep learning and updating your knowledge with new research and reviews that help you adjust your supplementation according to the latest available evidence.

Final Message

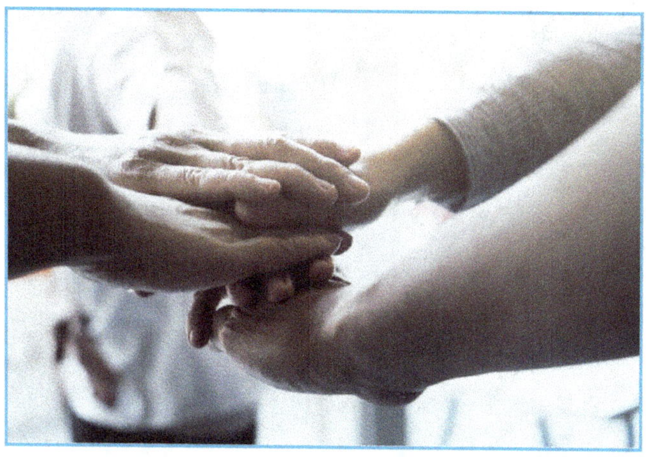

Before closing this book, I want to thank you for joining me on this journey toward a healthier, more balanced life. You have devoted time and effort to understanding how supplementation, along with exercise, nutrition, and rest, can transform your well-being. This path is not easy, but you've taken an important first step by investing in your knowledge and preparation.

Remember that every small change you make is a step forward toward your goals. The key lies in consistency, in maintaining a daily commitment to your health, and in listening to yourself and adjusting to what works best for you. Throughout this process, there will be days of progress and days of challenges, and in both moments, pushing forward is what will make the difference.

Never doubt your ability to achieve any goal you set for yourself. Trust in your discipline and in the power of your daily decisions. If something from this book has helped to strengthen your determination and guided you in better understanding your body and its needs, then this effort has been worthwhile.

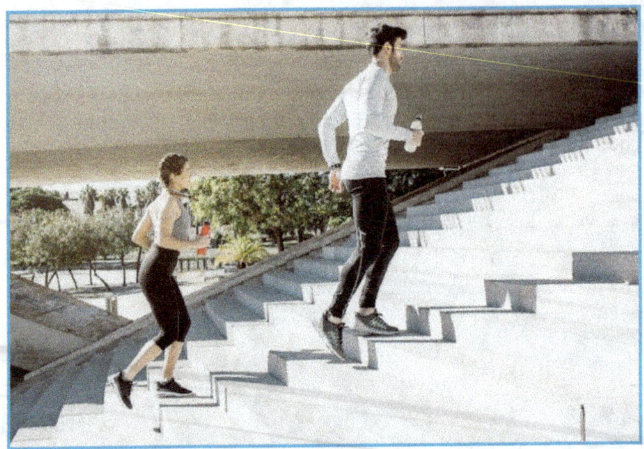

"Success is the sum of small efforts repeated day in and day out." — Robert Collier

With each step you take, you are closer to your best self. Move forward with confidence, and never underestimate the positive impact you are creating for your life!